The Fragile X Child

The Fragile X Child

Edited by
Betty B. Schopmeyer, MA, CCC-SLP
Speech-Language Pathologist
National Speech/Language Therapy Center
Rockville, Maryland
and
Fonda Lowe, MA, CCC-SLP
Speech-Language Pathologist
Ivymount School
Rockville, Maryland

SINGULAR PUBLISHING GROUP, INC.
San Diego, California

Singular Publishing Group, Inc.
4284 41st Street
San Diego, California 92105-1197

Typeset in 10/12 Palatino by House Graphics
Printed in the United States of America by McNaughton & Gunn

Library of Congress Cataloging-in-Publication Data
The Fragile X child / edited by Betty B. Schopmeyer and Fonda Lowe.
    p.   cm.
  Includes bibliographical references and index.
  ISBN 1-879105-83-7
  1. Fragile X syndrome—Patients—Rehabilitation. 2. Language
disorders in children—Patients—Rehabilitation. 3. Occupational
therapy for children.   I. Schopmeyer, Betty B. II. Lowe, Fonda.
  [DNLM: 1. Fragile X Syndrome. 2. Fragile X Syndrome—therapy.
3. Language Therapy—methods. 4. Occupational Therapy—methods.
5. Speech Therapy—methods. QS 677 F8104]
RJ506.F73F72 1992
616.85′88042—dc20
DNLM/DLC
for Library of Congress   92-17229
                                    CIP

CONTENTS

Contents

PREFACE

Many speech-language pathologists (SLPs) and occupational therapists (OTs) have children with fragile X syndrome in their caseloads and know little or nothing about the disorder. Because fragile X syndrome has only recently been identified as a major cause of inherited developmental delay, information is not yet widely available. Often clinicians first hear of fragile X when a child with this diagnosis appears in their therapy room. Also, children taken to a speech-language pathologist or occupational therapist because of delayed development may later be identified as having fragile X. Therapists need to learn about this syndrome for two reasons: to be able to knowledgeably treat children with fragile X and to be able to recommend testing for undiagnosed children exhibiting fragile X characteristics.

As SLPs and OTs may be the first professionals to be involved with a fragile X child and his family, this book is designed primarily for those clinicians. However, teachers, parents, and educational advocates will also find it helpful. Most information that is currently available about fragile X deals with its genetic and physical aspects. Speech and language therapy and occupational therapy are usually recommended, but there is little detailed information about the most effective therapeutic techniques to use. This book will assist therapists in recognizing, assessing, and planning treatment for children with fragile X syndrome.

The first section of this book, "What is Fragile X Syndrome?," provides an overview of background information necessary to understand the syndrome. Chapter 1 addresses the genetic aspects of fragile X and its unique and highly significant inheritance patterns. Dr. Black includes the most recent state-of-the-art developments in testing for fragile X, based on the recent discovery of the FMR-1 gene. Chapter 2, by one of the leaders in fragile X treatment and research, Dr. Randi Hagerman, explains the physical and medical profile of the fragile X child. Dr. Hagerman includes early development, medication, and the relationship of fragile X with autism.

Part II, "How Does the Child With Fragile X Function?," looks in detail at the characteristics of the child with fragile X in three areas. In Chapter 3, Dr. McClennen reviews the cognitive profile of the fragile X child, including assessment and learning style. Chapter 4 describes the fragile X sensory and motor characteristics critical to an understanding of the children's behavior. Ms. Anderson presents a pattern of typical strengths and weaknesses to help occupational therapists recognize the syndrome. In Chapter 5, Ms. Schopmeyer reviews the distinctive and unique speech and language characteristics typically seen in children with fragile X.

The third section, "How Do You Approach Intervention?," explains how to plan a program for and treat the child with fragile X in the areas of occupational therapy (Chapter 6), speech and language therapy (Chapter 7), and combined speech and language/ occupational therapy (Chapter 8). Ms. Lowe, Ms. Kaye, and Ms. Schopmeyer provide specific proposals for writing Individual Education Plans (IEPs), employing treatment techniques, and using practical materials. The chapter on combined treatment presents a novel approach to integrating occupational and speech and language therapy, including a rationale for using the model and a review of current literature. The treatment suggestions in Part III are drawn from clinical experience with many fragile X students at The Ivymount School in Rockville, MD, and from extensive review of the literature.

Part IV consists of a case study of a 7-year-old boy with fragile X syndrome. A thorough description, detailing how recommended treatment procedures were applied, is given of his first year at Ivymount School.

Appendix A provides a list of centers and organizations knowledgeable about fragile X syndrome.

Several decisions were made during the writing and editing of this book. The population of fragile X children addressed primarily includes boys between the ages of 3 and 12 years. The editors have chosen to limit discussion to this group because our experience has focused on these children. Girls with fragile X can also be affected; however, boys are typically more severely involved and are more homogeneous in their characteristics. The information presented can be modified and adapted to apply to girls with fragile X and also to other children who exhibit similar deficits in sensory integration and speech and language skills. The use of combined treatment is especially valuable for many children with neurological handicaps.

As the primary focus of the book is on boys with fragile X and because the majority of clinicians are usually female, "he" is used to refer to the child and "she" to refer to the therapists.

The editors have also decided not to address the controversy surrounding the efficacy of sensory integration treatment. Although proven results are not widely documented, much evidence exists supporting this treatment approach in certain populations, among them fragile X children. A list of references is provided following the references for Chapter 6, allowing interested readers to investigate sensory integration efficacy literature for themselves.

ACKNOWLEDGMENTS

We owe much to the superb staff of Ivymount School and to director Shari Gelman and assistant director Lillian Davis. Thank you for providing an atmosphere of constant learning, teaching, and support for new endeavors.

Special thanks to Linda and Dave Pender for their invaluable assistance in preparing the manuscript for this book.

CONTRIBUTORS

Sharon K. Anderson, OTR/L,
Neurodevelopmental Therapy
    Certified,
Sensory Integration and Praxis Test
    Certified
Coordinator of Occupational and
    Physical Therapy
Ivymount School
Rockville, Maryland

Susan H. Black, MD
Clinical Geneticist
Genetics & IVF Institute
Fairfax, Virginia

Randi J. Hagerman, MD
Developmental Pediatrician
The Children's Hospital Child
    Development Unit
Denver, Colorado

Sharon R. Kaye, OTR/L,
Occupational Therapist
Ivymount School
Rockville, Maryland

Fonda H. Lowe, MA, CCC-SLP
Speech-Language Pathologist
Ivymount School
Rockville, Maryland

Sandra E. McClennen, PhD
Psychologist, Department of Special
    Education
Eastern Michigan University
Ypsilanti, Michigan

Betty Schopmeyer, MA, CCC-SLP
Speech-Language Pathologist
National Speech/Language Therapy
    Center
Rockville, Maryland

PART I

WHAT IS FRAGILE X SYNDROME?

1

THE GENETICS OF FRAGILE X SYNDROME

The 1990s have been an exciting time for explanations of the genetic expression of a relatively common inherited disease called fragile X syndrome. It has long been recognized there are more retarded males than females in all populations. In 1974 a PhD thesis argued that this preponderance was due to X-linked genes (Lehrke, 1974). This definition of X-linked mental retardation (XLMR) had not been previously described because of a lack of obvious clinical findings in affected males. Once recognized, however, the category of nonspecific XLMR became important for classification of mental retardation, although it was recognized that this group was etiologically heterogeneous. Martin and Bell (1943) published one of the earliest pedigrees with XLMR.

Several other large family pedigrees were subsequently published. Dr. Herbert Lubs (1969) described a cytogenetic marker on the X chromosome (Figure 1-1) in four retarded males in a family with XLMR. This was thought to be isolated and no more attention was paid to it, but in 1973 another family was described with the same reported marker. However, as the report was in Portuguese, it largely went unnoticed! By the late 1970s it was recognized that a cytogenetic marker located on the end of the long arm of the X chromosome was not uncommon in some nonspecific X-linked mental retardation pedigrees. It took a cytogeneticist in Australia, Grant Sutherland (1977), to confirm the original observations by showing that the appearance of the marker depends on culturing

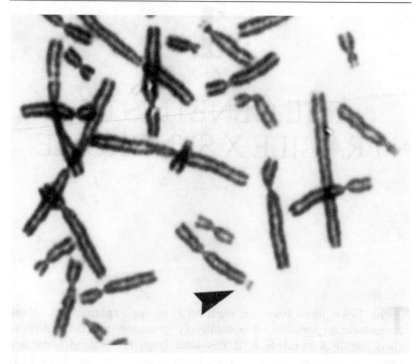

Figure 1-1. Human cell of unbanded chromosomes with ▶ denoting a fragile X q27.3 site. Courtesy of Dr. Patricia Howard-Peebles, Genetics & IVF Institute, Fairfax, Virginia.

cells under particular conditions. The condition needed is a tissue culture medium deficient in folic acid—the originally reported marker had disappeared because of the addition of folic acid as part of improvement in tissue culture techniques.

In addition, macroorchidism (large testes) had been observed in some patients with X-linked mental retardation. In 1978 another geneticist, Dr. Gillian Turner, and her co-workers showed that the macroorchidism was seen in some XLMR families also having the cytogenetic marker (Turner, Till, & Daniel, 1978). By 1982 the family members in the Martin-Bell pedigree were reevaluated and found to have the cytogenetic marker and macroorchidism. In recognition of this family, XLMR associated with the X chromosome marker was called the Martin-Bell syndrome. The "fragile X" designation came from the unique cytogenetic marker on the X chromosome. The syndrome is most commonly known by that designation now. Other early published XLMR pedigrees are negative for fragile X cytogenetically, indicating there are still X-linked genes for mental retardation yet to be defined.

Fragile X [fra(X)] syndrome is considered the most common inherited cause of mental retardation in males in the general population, with a calculated prevalance of 1 in 1,000 to 1 in 2,000. Only Down syndrome is seen more commonly but most Down syndrome is not inherited. Fra(X) syndrome has a significant impact on families, as it is always inherited. Therefore, the diagnosis of fragile X syndrome in a family often has counseling implications for multiple family members.

Since those initial clinical studies, a great deal of interest and scientific work has been done on fragile X syndrome, culminating in 1991 with the discovery of the fragile X gene. This has finally allowed for accurate carrier detection and prenatal testing for this important genetic disease. Discovery of the gene has also helped explain the distinctive and somewhat unique pattern of inheritance for this X-linked disease, which has been atypical in clinical presentation and inheritance. In order to understand how atypical fragile X syndrome is as an X-linked disease, however, it is necessary to first review how most diseases are inherited.

MENDELIAN MODES OF INHERITANCE

The human chromosome complement comprises 46 chromosomes: 22 pairs of homologous autosomes and one pair of sex chromosomes. Sixty thousand to 100,000 genes are contained in the human genome, the majority paired on autosomes and the two X chromosomes, if female. Autosomes are defined as the chromosomes that are not sex chromosomes. In females, the sex chromosomes should consist of two Xs, whereas males should have an X and a Y chromosome. Most of the genes on the X and the Y chromosome are not matched between themselves—this has important clinical significance in an X-linked pattern of inheritance that will be explained later. A gene mutation can occur at any locus (site) along the chromosome. Alleles are variations in genes at the same locus. A mutation in a gene is an abnormal gene structure that may or may not result in phenotypic (clinical) expression. Human genetic diseases are commonly inherited in three ways: autosomal dominant, autosomal recessive, and sex-linked. A brief description and diagram of each follows.

Autosomal Dominant Inheritance (Figure 1-2)

- A single mutation is sufficient to cause clinical effect.
- Males and females are equally at risk of inheriting the gene, as the mutation is found on an autosome.
- The risk in each pregnancy for offspring of an affected parent is 50% for inheriting the trait.

Two important genetic principles are observed in autosomal dominant inheritance: *penetrance and expressivity*. Penetrance defines whether someone carrying a mutant gene will show expression of that gene. There are some autosomal dominantly inherited diseases in which the penetrance is considered 100%—i.e., if the gene is being carried by that person, one will see clinical expression. Some dominant diseases have reduced penetrance. Because of this phenomenon, some family members may carry the gene without being affected, with "skipped" generations reported in the family. Expressivity defines the variability of clinical manifestations of a disease within multiple affected family members. Therefore, one may see family members with significant morbidity for the disease, whereas other family members may be only mildly affected.

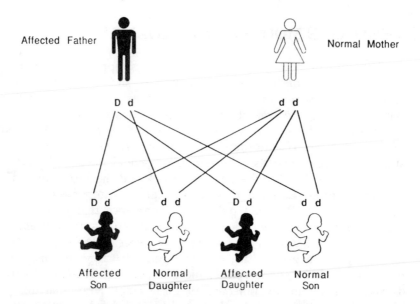

Figure 1-2. Autosomal dominant inheritance. D-dominant mutant gene on 1 homologous chromosome; d - normal gene at same locus on the other homologous chromosome. Pedigree courtesy of Greenwood Genetic Center, Greenwood, South Carolina.

A relatively common example of a dominant disease is neuro-fibromatosis (NF). NF is a neurocutaneous disorder that occurs in about 1 in 3,000 people in the general population. Patients may be seen clinically by speech-language pathologists, because learning disabilities have been increasingly recognized in affected patients. NF can present with symptoms ranging from skin markings called cafe-au-lait spots, which may be the only clinical manifestation, to significant intrabody tumors in the bone, brain, or heart, as well as disfiguring external skin tumors (neurofibromas) and other compli-cations. Within one family one may see all ranges of clinical expression. It is a disease with a high degree of penetrance, so that anyone carrying the gene will show some clinical manifestation, even if it is only five or six cafe-au-lait spots.

Dominant mutations may arise *denovo* in offspring. This happens with no previous family history, but the affected offspring will have a 50% risk for children to be affected with each pregnancy. It is also possible that a parent may have more than one germ cell (egg or sperm) with the same mutation present. This is called germ-line mosaicism. Parents who have germ-line mosaicism have a small increased risk of bearing other affected children, although the risk is not as high as the 50% in each pregnancy if a parent is carrying the mutation for the disease in "all cells."

Autosomal Recessive Inheritance (Figure 1-3)

- An affected offspring receives a double dose of a mutant gene.
- Carrier parents are clinically unaffected, although detec-tion of carrier status may be available through enzyme, DNA, or other specific marker analysis.
- Recurrence risk in each pregnancy is 25% if both parents are carriers.
- The risk of unaffected offspring being a carrier is 66% and being an unaffected, noncarrier is 33%.
- Males and females are at equal risk.

All people are thought to carry seven to eight recessive genes. Relatively common genetic diseases arising from autosomal recessive inheritance include cystic fibrosis in the white population, sickle cell disease in the black population, and Tay-Sachs disease in the Ash-kenazi Jewish population. A great deal of genetic research is focused on identification of carriers for autosomal recessive diseases, in order to provide appropriate genetic counseling. The risk for autosomal recessive diseases is higher in consanguinous matings. For example,

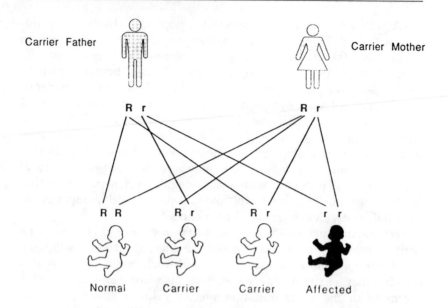

Figure 1-3. Autosomal recessive inheritance. R represents normal recessive gene on an autosome; r represents the mutant gene. Possible outcomes with each pregnancy. Courtesy of Greenwood Genetic Center, Greenwood, South Carolina.

first cousins share 1/8 of their genetic material in common and, therefore, are at higher risk of passing the same mutant gene to offspring. In the absence of a specific disease defined in first cousin marriages the empiric risk for birth defects is about 3% above general population risk (which in itself is about 3 to 4%). However, if an autosomal recessive inherited disease is diagnosed, the risk becomes 25% in each pregnancy. It must be emphasized, however, that the majority of autosomal recessive diseases are seen in families with no consanguinity or previous family history.

X-linked Inheritance (Figure 1-4)

- The cardinal rule for this mode of inheritance is that the trait may *not* be passed by the father to his son. A son should have inherited his father's Y chromosome.

- For a carrier mother, the risk in each pregnancy is: if a male, 50% risk of being affected and 50% risk of being unaffected; if a female, 50% risk of being a carrier and 50% chance of being a noncarrier.

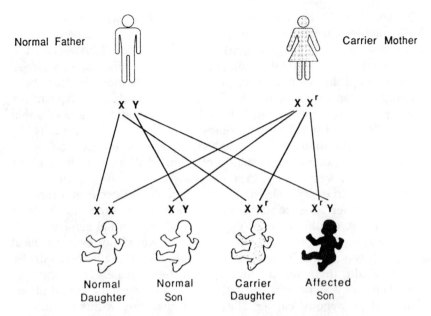

Figure 1-4. X-linked inheritance. X' represent the X-chromosome carrying a mutation; X represents the sex chromosome with the normal gene; Y is the male chromosome. Possible outcomes in each pregnancy. Pedigree courtesy of Greenwood Genetic Center, Greenwood, South Carolina.

- These disorders may be recessive or dominant. At present, X-linked dominant diseases are considered relatively uncommon. In those few that have been described, the inheritance of the gene in a male is considered lethal. Therefore, one will see a family history consistent with affected females, unaffected males, and perhaps a history of multiple miscarriages or stillborn males.

In some X-linked recessively inherited diseases, the birth of an affected male may arise from a new mutation occuring in the maternal germ cell. For example, in the X-linked muscle disorder, Duchenne muscular dystrophy (DMD), almost 1/3 of affected males have a *denovo* mutation in the DMD gene. This means the mother is not an obligate carrier of the disease. She may have germ-line mosaicism (more than one egg with mutations in the DMD gene), making her recurrence risk greater than the general population—but still relatively small. It is also unusual in typical X-linked inheritance for a carrier female to be affected. Because women have two X chromosomes, even if one X contains a recessive mutant gene, the other

X will "cover" for the mutation just as one sees in autosomal recessive disease carriers. An X-linked disease in a female could be manifest if she is homozygous for the mutation (she received a double dose of a mutant gene). For example, an offspring of a carrier for hemophilia who marries a male with hemophilia can bear daughters and sons at risk for hemophilia. Another mechanism for a carrier female to have an X-linked disease would be lack of some or all of one of her X chromosomes in body tissues. A Turner (45,X) female could manifest an X-linked disease. X inactivation is an important factor in manifestation of X-linked diseases in females. In such cases, very early in embryologic life, one of the Xs is inactivated in every cell. This inactivation should occur in a random manner; therefore, random inactivation of a "normal" X or a "mutant" X would allow for expression of the normal gene as much as the abnormal gene in a female and one would not expect clinical effect. If the normal X was randomly inactivated in a *majority* of cells, one would then see a clinically affected female. This principle explains why some women with normal chromosome constitutions and heterozygous carrier states will manifest X-linked disease. However, a female carrier with clinical expression of X-linked disease is still considered *the exception*, and not the rule.

Other modes of inheritance have been recently described that are themselves important, but are probably not relevant to fra(X) syndrome. If interested in further study, please refer to the selected genetics references at the end of the chapter.

FRAGILE X SYNDROME

With cytogenetic studies being available in fra (X) families, the atypical X-linked pattern of inheritance soon became apparent and the following patterns were defined in extended families:

1. Although one should have seen a 50% risk in each pregnancy of a carrier mother for affected males, the actual incidence of affected males in some generations was only 40%.
2. As many as 1/3 of carrier females could be affected with the learning disabilities, mental retardation, behavior disorders, and autistic-like behavior seen in affected males.
3. In clinically affected males and females expression of the fragile site could be demonstrated in only 3 to 50% of peripheral blood cells. The percentage of positive cells would depend on the age when the blood was taken. In obligate carrier females, the cytogenetic percentage of expression of

the fra(X) site would decrease over time—therefore making it less likely that one could confirm carrier status in an older woman than in a younger obligate carrier female. Almost 50% of carrier females would also be cytogenetically negative.

4. The frequency and severity of fra(X) syndrome increased from generation to generation.

5. It became apparent that there were males who were "silent carriers," now known as normal transmitting males. These males made up the 10% of the theoretical 50% risk for carrier mothers. These family members would be cytogenetically negative and normal clinically: All biological daughters would be obligate carriers, as they could only receive an X from their fathers. The daughters of normal transmitting males would again be clinically normal and cytogenetically negative, but then would be at risk of affected offspring.

A pedigree illustrating the inheritance pattern of a multigenerational fragile X family is seen in Figure 1-5. From this family pedigree, one can see the increasing risk and clinical severity through the generations. There is also a higher risk of affected offspring if one is cytogenetically positive and/or clinically affected.

An important limitation of the cytogenetic testing in fra(X) syndrome was that 50% of obligate carrier females would be cytogenetically negative. Thus female relatives of affected family members would often be faced with uncertainty about their status as carriers, because accurate carrier status could not be provided. Similarly, some clinically normal males in fra(X) families would be carriers, but their status could not be defined cytogenetically. For these normal transmitting males, grandchildren would be at risk, because all their daughters would be obligate carriers, but also unaffected. This "skipping" of two generations in a family would for most other X-linked disorders mean there was little subsequent risk of affected offspring, but this is not true for fra(X) syndrome.

Rapid advances in molecular genetics began to provide more information in multigenerational families. Until 1991, the techniques used in fragile X families involved DNA linkage analysis. Again, because of limitations of this book's scope, specific discussion about techniques for processing and analyzing DNA cannot be detailed. The listed genetics references review this information.

Linkage analysis consists of using enzymes called restriction endonucleases to cut DNA segments as closely linked to the gene of interest as possible. One then compares the pattern of the "cut"

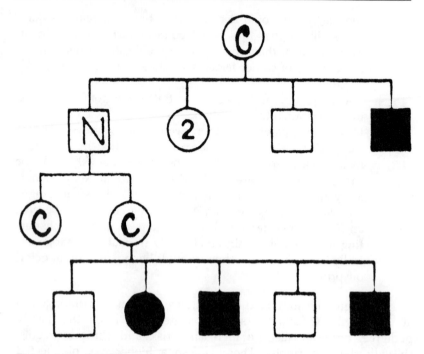

Figure 1-5. A fragile X pedigree. N - normal transmitting male; C - carrier female; 2 - 2 daughters; ● ■ - affected. Courtesy of Patricia Howard-Peebles. Genetics & IVF Institute, Fairfax, Virginia.

DNA segments of affected family members with the DNA patterns of other extended family members to define who is at risk for being a carrier or a normal transmitting male in fragile X syndrome. There were significant limitations in using this diagnostic technique: the most important being that the linkage analysis was often *not* informative. Another general limitation of DNA linkage analysis was that it does not identify genotype within a family so it couldn't be used to confirm or rule out the diagnosis in family members with a few or questionable clinical findings. For several years, however, both cytogenetic and DNA linkage analysis were recommended for prenatal testing in at-risk families. As techniques were combined, the accuracy of predicting outcomes was greatly improved.

The Molecular Genetic Defect in Fragile X Syndrome

For years, scientists and clinicians have tried to understand why the cytogenetic expression of the fra(X)q27.3 site on the X-chromosome was indicative of clinical disease. There are other fragile sites known on human chromosomes, but none of the others have been associated with clinical disease. In 1991 several groups working simultaneously in different laboratories described the gene responsible for fragile X syndrome, which is now called fragile X mental retardation-1 (FMR—1) gene (Rousseau, Heitz, Oberle, & Mandel, 1991; Verkerk et al., 1991). However, the *function* of this gene is still not known. So, even as we have begun to understand on a molecular basis the clinical (phenotypic) expression of the disease, we do not yet understand what this gene does. Presently, the predicted protein within the FMR-1 gene has no equivalent structure pattern with known proteins.

The FMR-1 gene has sequences that span over 80 kilobases (80,000 bases), with messenger RNA of 4.8 kilobases (4,800 bases) that is expressed in the human brain, lymphocytes, and placenta. There is a lengthy cytidine-guanosine-guanosine (CGG) trinucleotide repeat within the gene that produces multiple arginine (an amino acid) residues. In normal people there are usually 15 to 65 copies of this $(CGG)°$ triplet (mean range is around 40). The fragile X mutation is an increase in the number of these $(CGG)°$ repeats in the FMR-1 gene. The normal X chromosome will carry a variable but supposedly stable number of these repeats ranging, as we discussed, from 15 to about 50 triplets (45 to 150 bases). When these $(CGG)°$ repeats begin to increase in size (50 to 200) it now becomes a premutation (or a small insert). This premutation is what is seen in normal transmitting males and remains unchanged during spermatogenesis. When inherited by a female, the premutation may increase in size during oogenesis. When the premutation increases in size until it is 600 bases or greater [200 sets of $(CGG)°$], it becomes the "full" mutation that is associated with the disease phenotype. In addition, in the human genome, when a gene or mutant gene becomes a certain length, methyl groups are attached. Methylation of a gene usually means that that length of DNA will *not* be transcribed by messenger RNA, so one does *not see expression of that gene* or part of a gene. Experimental work showing this lack of expression when the "full" mutation of the FMR-1 gene is present has already been demonstrated.

A diagram of the direct DNA analysis for the FMR-1 gene using Mandel probes is found in Figure 1-6. This represents a Southern blot analysis for DNA. Enzymes are used to cut the FMR-1 gene at specific sites. In the active normal X, the cut site will give a DNA fragment length of 2.8 kilobases. In the inactive X (which has been methylated) the enzyme won't recognize the usual enzyme site, so a 5.2 kilobase fragment will be seen. As you might expect, therefore,

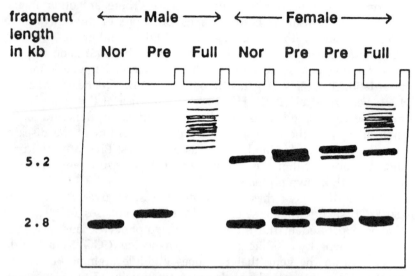

Figure 1-6. Schematic Diagram of Direct DNA analysis of FMR-1 gene (Mandel method). Nor - normal; pre - premutation; full - full mutation; kb - kilobases. Courtesy of Dr. Anne Maddalena, Genetics & IVF Institute, Fairfax, Virginia.

in males you will see only one fragment length (the 2.8 kilobase in a normal X, for example); in females, who have two Xs, you will see two fragment lengths, the density of which may vary, depending on the randomization of X inactivation. Please refer back to this diagram as needed. The different DNA patterns seen in fragile X families will be explained in detail.

Normal Transmitting Males

Normal transmitting males in fragile X families will show a mutation by an increased length of the CGG repeat, but the increase in size is about 50 to 100 triplets (150 to 600 bases)—so only a single band slightly higher than the normal 2.8 kilobase fragment will be seen. This is called the premutation. In family studies, these larger fragments are all inherited either unchanged or during oogenesis by the daughters of normal transmitting males, and there is an increase or decrease in size of 50 to 100 triplets (150 to 300 bases). The $(CGG)°$ associated with FMR-1 in normal transmitting males usually remains unmethylated and is transcribed as in normal males.

Carrier Females

When looking at obligate carrier females, one will see an abnormal fragment length on DNA analysis, regardless of expression of the fragile site cytogenetically. As noted, almost 50% of obligate carrier females will not express the fragile site on cytogenetic analysis. Carrier females or obligate carrier females of normal transmitting males will usually show two normal DNA fragments (2.8 and 5.2 kilobases) and two fragments that are 50 to 200 triplets (150 to 600) base pairs larger than normal. Females with fragile X expression cytogenetically and phenotypically have "full" mutations, so there is a large band or a "smear" representing multiple fragments. After direct DNA analysis of multiple fra(X) families, carrier females whose DNA shows premutations (a small increase in size of the gene) do not appear to have clinical expression of fragile X. However, not *all* females with large fragments or smears on DNA analysis will express the fragile X site cytogenetically or be clinically affected with behavior disorders, mental retardation, or severe learning disabilities. It is likely that the presence of the normal X (if active) modifies clinical expression of the disease. A carrier mother with a full mutation (large fragment) may have affected sons who have either smaller or larger DNA fragments (premutations—full mutations). It appears that significant change in size of the DNA fragment for the FMR-1 gene can occur during oogenesis.

Clinically Affected Males With Fragile X Syndrome

In clinically affected males with fragile X syndrome, an increase of 1 to 4 kilobases (1,000 to 4,000 bases) is seen usually in the absence of the 2.8-kilobase DNA fragment. The affected males will show multiple larger discrete bands or a faint smear of larger fragments on the Southern blot. In some affected males, a normal size band with the full mutation is seen. This likely represents mosaicism (presence of more than one cell line) in different body tissues. Mosaicism is seen in other cytogenetic diseases such as Down syndrome. The presence of the normal cell line may modify the clinical picture. The rare fragile X cytogenetic positive patients have not shown the characteristic CGG length mutation: their clinical disease has been considered atypical for fragile X syndrome and their fragile X cytogenetic expression low.

Therefore, in summary:

1. Fragile X syndrome is an X-linked genetic disorder. There is cytogenetic expression of a fragile site at Xq27.3. The FMR-1 gene is also located at this site on the X chromosome.

2. The mothers of affected children are always carriers. Sporadic full mutations have not yet been observed.
3. The larger the DNA insertion (increase in CGG repeat size) a woman carries, the greater the chance that her children will be clinically affected.
4. A boy who inherits a "full" mutation will be affected.
5. A girl who inherits a "full" mutation *may* be affected.
6. The identification of the DNA gene mutation seen in fragile X explains the atypical pattern of X-linked inheritance.

However, there is still a great deal to be accomplished with fragile X syndrome. A gene associated with clinical expression of the disease has been identified, but its function is not yet known. Continued research is needed to identify functions of this gene, because specific treatments and gene therapy will then be possible. In the meantime, identification of fragile X syndrome in children and adults who present with learning disabilities, mental retardation, and behavior disorders continues to be important, because of the inherited nature of the disease. Fragile X testing should be considered for all males and even females who present with learning disorders, autistic-like behavior, and other behavioral problems in the absence of any other known specific etiology. Although the presence of a specific family history of X-linked male mental retardation is important, testing should be considered independently of such a history, especially if the clinical picture of the presenting patient suggests fragile X syndrome.

REFERENCES

Lehrke, R.G. (1974). X-linked mental retardation and verbal disability. *Birth Defects, 10*, 1-100.

Lubs, H.A. (1969). A marker X chromosome. *American Journal of Human Genetics, 21*, 231-244.

Martin, J.P., & Bell, J. (1943). A pedigree of mental defect showing sex-linkage. *Journal of Neurology and Psychiatry, 6*, 154-157.

Rousseau, F., Heitz, D., Oberlé, I., & Mandel, J-L. (1991). Selection in blood cells from female carriers of the fragile X syndrome: Inverse correlation between age and proportion of active X chromosomes carrying the full mutation. *Journal of Medical Genetics, 28*, 830-836.

Sutherland, G.R. (1977). Fragile sites on human chromosomes: Demonstration of their dependence on the type of tissue culture medium. *Science, 197*, 265-266.

Turner, G., Till, R., & Daniel, A. (1978). Marker X chromosome, mental retardation and macro-orchidism. *New England Journal of Medicine, 303*, 662-664.

Verkerk, A.J.M., Pieretti, M., Sutcliffe, J.S., Fu, Y.H., Kuhl, D.P.A., Pizzuti, A., Reiner, O., Richards, S., Victoria, M.F., Zhang, F., Eussen, B.E., van Ommen, G.J.B., Blonden, L.A.J., Riggins, G.J., Chastain, J.L., Kunst, C.B., Galjaard, H., Caskey, C.T., Nelson, D.L., Oostra, B.A., & Warren, S.T. (1991). Identification of a gene (FMR-1) containing a CGG repeat coincident with a breakpoint cluster region exhibiting length variation in fragile X sydrome. *Cell, 65,* 905-914.

ADDITIONAL READINGS

Connor, J.M. (1991). Cloning of the gene for the fragile X syndrome: Implications for the clinical geneticist. *Journal of Medical Genetics, 28,* 811-813.

Hagerman, R.J., & Silverman, A.S. (1991). *Fragile X syndrome: Diagnosis, treatment, and research.* Baltimore: The Johns Hopkins University Press.

Hirst, M.C., Nakahori, Y., Knight, S.J.L., Schwartz, C., Thibodeau, S.N., Roche, A., Flint, T.J., Connor, J.M., Fryns, J-P., & Davies, K.E. (1991). Genotype prediction in the fragile X syndrome. *Journal of Medical Genetics, 28,* 824-829.

Jackson, J.F. (1991). *Genetics and you.* Jackson, MI: Fenwick Press.

Nora, J.J., & Fraser, F.C. (1989). *Medical genetics: Principles and Practice* (3rd Ed.). Philadelphia & London: Lea & Febiger.

Pergolizzi, R.G., Erster, S.H., Goonewardena, P., & Brown, W.T. (1992, February). Detection of full fragile X mutation. *The Lancet, 339,* 271-272.

Poustka, A., Dietrich, A., Langenstein, G., Toniolo, D., Warren, S.T., & Lehrach, H. (1991). Physical map of human Xq27-qter: Localizing the region of the fragile X mutation. Proceedings of the National Academy of Science, USA. *Genetics, 88,* 8302-8306.

Rousseau, F., Heitz, D., Biancalana, V., Blumenfield, S., Kretz, C., Boue, J., Tommerup, N., Van Der Hagen, C., DeLozier-Blanchet, C., Croquette, M-F., Gilgenkrantz, S., Jalbert, P., Voelckel, M-A., Oberlé, I., & Mandel, J-L. (1991). Direct diagnosis by DNA analysis of the fragile X syndrome of mental retardation. *The New England Journal of Medicine, 325,* 1673-1681.

Shapiro, L.R., (1991, December 12). The fragile X syndrome: A peculiar pattern of inheritance. *The New England Journal of Medicine,* 1736-1737.

Thompson, J.S., & Thompson, M.W. (1986). *Genetics in medicine* (4th Ed.). Philadelphia: W.B. Saunders Company.

Vincent, A., Heitz, D., Petit, C., Kretz, C., Oberlé, I., & Mandel, J.L. (1991). Abnormal pattern detected in fragile-X patients by pulsed-field gel electrophoresis. *Nature, 349,* 624-626.

Webb, T. (1991). Molecular genetics of fragile X: A cytogenetics viewpoint. Report of the Fifth International Symposium on X-Linked Mental Retardation, Strasbourg, France, August 12-16, 1991 (organizer Dr. J-L Mandel). *Journal of Medical Genetics, 28,* 814-817.

2

MEDICAL ASPECTS OF THE FRAGILE X SYNDROME

The fragile X syndrome is the most common known inherited cause of mental retardation. Although first identified in 1969, very few individuals were diagnosed in the United States during the 1970s. Through the work of Dr. Gillian Turner in Australia and Dr. Pat Howard-Peebles in the United States (Turner, 1973) the clinical phenotype became more readily recognized in the 1980s. The frequency of diagnosis has increased quite dramatically during the last decade and will now be simplified by the use of DNA technology. The spectrum of involvement has expanded to not only include mental retardation but also learning disability with a normal IQ in mildly affected individuals and emotional or behavioral problems.

Individuals with fragile X syndrome usually present with language delays and behavioral problems, particularly hyperactivity. As infants they may be irritable and difficult to cuddle because of tactile defensiveness. Often unusual hand movements, such as hand-flapping or hand-biting, develop in early childhood, and tantrum behavior is common. On examination, young fragile X boys are usually hypotonic with hyperextensible finger joints. The thumb can be double-jointed, and the skin usually has a soft velvety texture so that the palms are often wrinkled. Because of motor delays and hypotonia the occupational therapist or the physical therapist may be the first person to assess a fragile X child—even before the diagnosis is made.

In fragile X men, the most distinguishing physical features are long or prominent ears, a long, narrow face, and large testicles or macroorchidism. These features, however, are often absent in pre-pubertal children. Therefore, the behavioral features are the most helpful for diagnosis.

BEHAVIOR AND LANGUAGE

The behavioral features in early childhood usually include poor eye contact in approximately 90% of the youngsters and tactile defensiveness in the majority. Fragile X children usually have problems with a short attention span, distractibility, and impulsivity often associated with hyperactivity in the majority of boys. Language development is almost always delayed and lack of significant speech at 2 1/2 or 3 years of age is a common presenting feature. In addition, there may be unusual aspects to their speech such as perseveration, which is seen in more than 90% of the children. This will usually be manifested by repeating a word or asking the same question over and over again, even when the word is responded to or the question adequately answered.

Fragile X children also have difficulty in making transitions— that is, moving from one activity to another. They are easily over-whelmed by environmental stimuli, such as visual or auditory information. When they are frustrated or overstimulated, tantrum behavior often occurs. This problem is most commonly seen in shopping centers, grocery stores, or in crowds where there is a lot of activity.

Fragile X and Autism

Because of the unusual behavioral features seen in fragile X syndrome, there has been significant study of the association between fragile X and autism. The majority of fragile X boys will demonstrate autistic-like features, such as poor eye contact, tactile defensiveness, perseveration, hand-flapping, hand-biting, or other unusual hand stereotypies. However, the majority of fragile X children are interested in relating socially. The combination of autistic-like features and sociability leads to an approach-withdrawal behavior in social interactions. For instance, Wolff, Gardner, Paccia, and Lappen (1989) have reported that the greeting behavior of a fragile X male includes the extension of the hand into a handshake; however, there is a turning of the body away from the person who is greeted. Eye contact is also avoided. Because of difficulty in tolerating sensory stimuli, most fragile X children are diagnosed with a sensory motor integration (SI) deficit. Treatment of SI problems can be helpful for behavioral problems, including hyperactivity and aggression in fragile X individuals and will be discussed in detail in other chapters.

Approximately 15% of fragile X male children or adults will demonstrate the full syndrome of autism. Autism is more common in individuals with severe cognitive deficits. When autistic males are screened with cytogenetic testing, approximately 7% will turn out to have fragile X syndrome. Autism has also been described in fragile X girls, although the vast majority of females who demonstrate the fragile X chromosome do not have autism. Females with fragile X more commonly have shyness and social anxiety. In addition, one-third of fragile X-positive girls will have attention deficit disorder with or without hyperactivity.

PHYSICAL FEATURES

Approximately 80% of adult fragile X males will have large or prominent ears, a long face, and macroorchidism, or large testicles. The testicles of an adult fragile X male usually vary from 40 ml to 80 ml in volume, which is two to three times the normal testicular volume. However, large testicles and a long, narrow face are more common after puberty than before puberty. Younger fragile X children more typically present with prominent ears and hyperextensible finger joints. Figures 2-1, 2-2, 2-3, and 2-4 show boys with fragile X syndrome at various ages. Flat feet, pectus excavatum, and a high-arched palate are also common. These features are consistent with a connective tissue dysplasia, although the structural abnormality is not known. Waldstein et al. (1986) reported abnormal elastin fibers in the skin of fragile X males compared to controls, but further studies have not been carried out. Mitral valve prolapse (MVP) is also common in fragile X males and is thought to be related to the connective tissue problems. The MVP is usually recognized by a click or murmur on cardiac examination. Echocardiography will document prolapse of the mitral valve and, on occasion, a more significant murmur secondary to mitral regurgitation (blood moving back through the mitral valve instead of out through the aorta as the ventricles contract) will be heard.

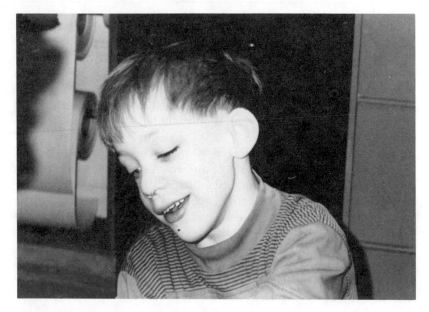

Figure 2-1. A 6-year-old boy with fragile X syndrome.

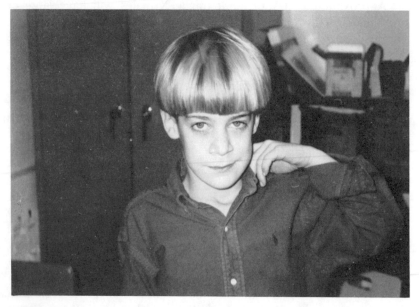

Figure 2-2. A 9 year old.

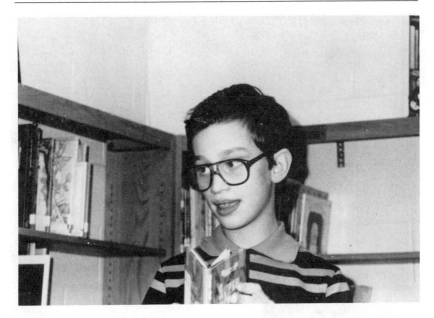

Figure 2-3. An 11 year old.

The loose connective tissue in fragile X patients on rare occasion may lead to problems, such as hernias or joint dislocation. Perhaps the connective tissue dysplasia, in addition to the facial structural changes, leads to the very frequent history of recurrent otitis media in young fragile X boys. This is a problem for about 60% of individuals and usually requires aggressive treatment and placement of polyethylene (PE) tubes to normalize hearing. This treatment is important to improve language development which is already compromised by the fragile X syndrome. Other medical problems, such as scoliosis, or more significant malformations, such as club foot anomaly or cleft palate, are occasionally seen in fragile X.

Ophthalmological problems are common in fragile X children and strabismus is seen in approximately 35%. Strabismus, or a weak eye muscle, usually manifests by one eye turning in or out, particularly when the child is tired. This requires a prompt ophthalmological assessment and treatment which may include patching, glasses, or surgery. Nystagmus (quick lateral movements of the eye), ptosis (eyelid drooping), and nearsightedness or farsightedness are also seen more frequently in fragile X children than in the general population. It is important for all fragile X children to be evaluated by an ophthalmologist or optometrist before 4 or 5 years of age. As

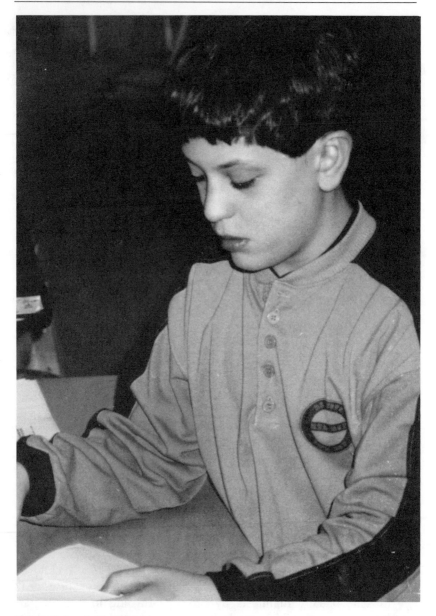

Figure 2-4.   A 12 year old.

the examination may be difficult because of poor child cooperation, more than one visit is sometimes necessary to complete the evaluation.

Approximately 20% of fragile X children have seizures. The seizures may include short staring spells, partial motor seizures, or grand mal episodes. Seizures need to be evaluated with an EEG and usually require treatment with anticonvulsant medication, such as carbamazepine (Tegretol). Brain imaging studies have demonstrated abnormalities, including enlarged ventricles often associated with a large head circumference. Studies by Reiss, Patel, Kumar, and Freund (1988) have documented a small posterior cerebellar vermis in both fragile X males and females as compared to controls. The hypoplasia of the vermis is thought to be related to the sensory integration problems common in this disorder.

Females With Fragile X

Only 50% of females who carry the fragile X gene may be cyto-genetically positive; that is, on chromosomal testing demonstrate the fragile X chromosome. Females who carry the fragile X gene but do not demonstrate the fragile X chromosome cytogenetically are usually unaffected physically and intellectually. Fragile X positive girls, on the other hand, will show a spectrum of involvement ranging from learning disability with a normal IQ to mental retardation. Approximately 25% of fragile X positive girls will have an IQ below 70 and an additional 25% will have an IQ in the borderline intellectual range. Of the 50% of fragile X girls who have a normal IQ, approximately one-half will require special education help in school. Math deficits, language delays, sensory integration problems, and attentional problems are common difficulties for fragile X positive girls. In general, fragile X girls are less affected than fragile X boys, because they have two X chromosomes with only one of the X chromosomes carrying the fragile X mutation.

TREATMENT

The approach to treatment of the fragile X syndrome involves a variety of professionals and a multimodality approach. Most fragile X boys and significantly affected girls require special education help, speech and language therapy, occupational therapy, physical therapy, and medical intervention. This section will focus on medication that can be helpful for behavioral problems or medical complications in fragile X. Medications, however, should always be used in conjunction with other interventions to optimize outcome. There is currently no cure for fragile X.

The majority of young fragile X boys and a significant percentage of affected fragile X girls suffer from attentional problems and impulsivity, which can occur in conjunction with hyperactivity. Speech and language therapy and occupational therapy can address the issues and improve the problems. In addition, medical intervention can also be helpful. Folic acid was the first medication used to treat attentional problems and its use has been controversial. Several reports have described no effect from folic acid, and other reports have described a significant improvement in attention and concentration, particularly in young children. In my experience, approximately 50% of young fragile X children improve with folic acid and it can be tried at a young age. Folic acid has been previously used in a dose of 1 mg per kg up to 10 mg per day. I recommend a trial of folic acid for a 2- to 3-month period and careful documentation of any improvement in attention, concentration, or language development. If it is not helpful, it can be discontinued. If it is helpful for the child, it can be continued; however, follow-up medical studies should include blood work, at least annually (Hagerman & Silverman, 1991).

Stimulant medication, including methylphenidate (Ritalin), dextroamphetamine (Dexedrine), or pemoline (Cylert) have been effective for approximately two-thirds of hyperactive fragile X children. The side effects of stimulant medication include cardiovascular stimulation and appetite suppression. Fragile X children also appear to be more sensitive to stimulant medication than other hyperactive children and can more readily have difficulty with irritability, temper tantrums, and mood lability. If side effects become a significant problem, stimulant medication should be discontinued. If stimulant medication is recommended by a physician, it should be started at a low dose, trial basis with careful follow-up.

There are a variety of medications that can be used to treat attentional problems and impulsivity in lieu of stimulant medication. These options include clonidine (Catapres), which is an antihypertensive medication that also improves attention and concentration. The main side effect is sleepyness and, again, it should be started at a low dose and followed carefully by a physician. In addition, Imipramine (Tofranil), which is a tricyclic antidepressant, has been used in fragile X for treatment of attentional problems or hyperactivity. It is also effective in treating enuresis or bed-wetting. Its side effects include cardiovascular stimulation and the slowing of cardiac conduction at higher doses. Approximately 50% of fragile X children have had an adverse response to Imipramine, with an increase in aggressive behavior or tantrums. Thioridazine (Mellaril) has also been used in the treatment of hyperactivity or behavior problems in fragile X. It is a major tranquilizer and an antipsychotic medication. Antipsychotic medication can cause a variety of long-term side effects, including unusual motor movements. However, this has rarely been seen in fragile X patients when thioridazine is used at a low dose. Significant psychotic ideation that occasionally occurs in fragile X patients requires antipsychotic medication for optimal treatment.

Aggression may become a difficulty, particularly close to adolescence, or in adulthood. A variety of medications have been used effectively for treatment of aggression and these include fluoxetine (Prozac), lithium, beta blockers, and thioridazine (Mellaril). It is important to remember that treatment of aggression or other behavior problems should include a professional team and intervention such as counseling, sensory integration therapy including calming techniques, behavior modification, and enhanced structure in the environment. Psychotherapy or counseling has been underutilized for mentally retarded individuals, yet it can be very effective in dealing with aggression or other behavior problems.

GENETICS

An important reason to make the diagnosis of fragile X syndrome is recognition of the genetic aspect of the disorder. Because it is carried on the X chromosome, 50% of the offspring of a carrier mother will inherit the gene. Therefore, siblings of the diagnosed child and future children are at very high risk of suffering from learning disabilities or mental retardation. If the carrier mother inherited the gene from her father, then all of his female offspring are also carriers, although it cannot pass from father to son. It is essential that a detailed family history be reviewed, preferably by a genetics counselor, so that individuals who are at risk of carrying the gene or are affected by fragile X syndrome undergo genetic testing for diagnosis and treatment. After diagnosis, the family should be put in touch with a local parent support group. The family or the clinician can contact the National Fragile X Foundation at 1-800-688-8765 to find a resource center or parent support group nearest to them. (See Appendix A.)

In the summer of 1991, the fragile X mental retardation gene (FMR-1) was sequenced (Verkerk et al., 1991) and several laboratories (Rousseau et al., 1991; Verkerk et al., 1991; Yu, Pritchard, & Kremer, 1991) identified an unstable CGG nucleotide sequence at the gene site. In affected individuals, the CGG sequence can lengthen to several hundred or 1,000 CGG repeats, whereas carriers who are unaffected have from 50 to 200 repetitions of the CGG repeat. Normal individuals who do not carry the mutation have less than 50 CGG repeats. It is unknown why the CGG repeats can lengthen from one generation to another. When the length becomes excessive (greater than 200 repeats), the normal FMR-1 protein is not produced and it is the lack of this protein that causes the fragile X syndrome.

Presently, there are many centers studying the relationship between fragile X molecular findings and the physical and intellectual phenotype. The new advances in the molecular field will lead to a better understanding of the syndrome and new insights into treatment.

REFERENCES

Hagerman, R.J., & Silverman, A.C. (1991). *Fragile X syndrome: Diagnosis, treatment and research.* Baltimore: The Johns Hopkins University Press.

Lubs, H.A. (1969). A marker X chromosome. *American Journal of Human Genetics, 21,* 231-234.

Reiss, A.L., Patel, S., Kumar, A.J., & Freund, L. (1988). Preliminary communication: Neuroanatomical variations of the posterior fossa in men with the fragile X (Martin-Bell) syndrome. *American Journal of Medical Genetics, 31,* 407-414.

Rousseau, F., Heitz, D., Biancalana, V., Blumenfield, S., Kretz, C., Boue, J., Tommerup, N., Van Der Hagen, C., DeLozier-Blanchet, C., Croquette, M-F., Gilgenkrantz, S., Jalbert, P., Voelckel, M-A, Oberle, I., & Mandel, J-L. (1991). Direct diagnosis by DNA analysis of the fragile X syndrome of mental retardation. *New England Journal of Medicine, 325,* 1673-1681.

Turner, G. (1973). Historical overview of X-linked mental retardation. In R.J. Hagerman and P.M. McBogg (Eds.) *Fragile X syndrome: Diagnosis, biochemistry, and intervention* (pp. 1-16). Dillon CO: Spectra Publishing.

Verkerk, A.J.M., Pieretti, M., Sutcliffe, J.S., Fu, Y.H., Kuhl, D.P.A., Pizzuti, A., Reiner, O., Richards, S., Victoria, M.F., Zhang, F., Eussen, B.E., van Ommen, G.J.B., Blonden, L.A.J., Riggins, G.J., Chastain, J.L., Kunst, C.B., Galjaard, H., Caskey, C.T., Nelson, D.L., Oostra, B.A., & Warren, S.T. (1991). Identification of a gene (FMR-1) containing a CGG repeat coincident with a breakpoint cluster region exhibiting length variation in fragile X syndrome. *Cell, 65,* 905-914.

Waldstein, G., Mierau, G., Ahmad, R., Thibodeau, S.N., Hagerman, R.J., & Caldwell, S. (1986). Fragile X syndrome: Skin elastin abnormalities. In E.F. Gilbert and J.M. Opitz (Eds.) *Genetic aspects of developmental pathology* (pp. 103-114). New York: Alan R. Lis.

Wolff, P.H., Gardner, J., Paccia, J.J., & Lappen, J. (1989). The greeting behavior of fragile X males. *American Journal of Mental Retardation, 93,* 406-411.

Yu, S., Pritchard, M., Kremer, E., et al. (1991). Fragile X genotype characterized by an unstable region of DNA. *Science, 252,* 1179-1181.

ADDITIONAL READINGS

Brown, W.T., Jenkins, E.C., & Cohen, I.L., (1986). Fragile X and autism: A multicenter survey. *American Journal of Medical Genetics, 23,* 341-352.

Brown, W.T., Jenkins, E.C., & Neri, G., (1991). Conference report: 4th International workshop on the fragile X and X-linked mental retardation. *American Journal of Medical Genetics, 38,* 158-172.

Davies, K.E. (Ed.). (1989). *Fragile X syndrome.* New York: Oxford University Press.

Hagerman, R.J., Amiri K., & Cronister, A. (1991). The fragile X checklist. *American Journal of Medical Genetics, 38,* 283-287.

Hagerman, R.J., Jackson, C., Amiri, K., Cronister, A., Wittenberger, M., Schreiner, R., & Sobesky, W. (in press). Fragile X girls: Physical and neurocognitive status and outcome. *Pediatrics.*

PART II

HOW DOES THE CHILD WITH FRAGILE X FUNCTION?

3

COGNITIVE CHARACTERISTICS, ASSESSMENT, AND INTERVENTION IN FRAGILE X SYNDROME

Children with fragile X syndrome present a unique and fascinating pattern of cognitive, behavioral, and affective characteristics. What you think you see is not what you get. Hidden beneath the challenging and often puzzling behaviors caused by central nervous system dysfunction are skills in visual learning, surprising evidence of memory and understanding, a sense of humor, and affection for and need of other people. These are particularly vulnerable children who require skilled assistance based on understanding of their situation in order to express their hidden capabilities.

This chapter will first address the cognitive characteristics of males. Information from standardized testing and a discussion of reported intelligence test score changes with age is followed by descriptions of cognitive strengths and weaknesses in areas that have been identified in the literature and in practice. When possible, specific suggestions are made for restructuring or adapting tasks. Then the available information about cognitive characteristics of females is reported. Addressing both males and females, a section on assessment discusses formal and informal assessment and interpretation of results in light of current knowledge and recommends instruments for intelligence testing. The last section, covering learning style, suggests ways that interventions and decisions about school placement can build on knowledge of cognitive characteristics in order to maximize learning opportunities for children with fragile X syndrome.

A neuropsychology of fragile X syndrome is only beginning to be studied and defined. However, it is clear that fragile X syndrome has implications for both cognitive and behavioral characteristics. While cognition and behavior may be artificially separated for descriptive purposes, in reality they interact. The behaviors that children exhibit based on their neurology influence their cognitive characteristics. The ways in which children cognitively understand the world around them in turn influence their behavior. Thus, as cognitive characteristics are discussed, there are references to interactions with behavioral characteristics.

Males' and females' profiles of both behavioral characteristics and of cognitive strengths and weaknesses are distinctive enough to require separate descriptions, although there are areas of overlap. As a group, males demonstrate many more deficits than females. They have, therefore, been brought to professional attention more frequently and earlier in their lives and have consequently been studied more than females.

The behavioral characteristics most relevant to a discussion of cognitive characteristics center on central nervous system dysfunction and the inability of the brain to fully process and/or organize the flow of sensory impulses (discussed in Chapter 4). Hypersensitivity to visual, auditory, olfactory, and tactile stimuli is common. Boys with fragile X syndrome frequently present with hyperactivity and attention deficit disorder (ADHD) and the related characteristics of distractibility, impulsivity, and a high level of anxiety. Behaviors such as hand biting and flapping, gaze avoidance, tactile defensiveness, and perseverative speech are also typical and show a marked increase at times of higher anxiety. Hagerman (1991) has suggested that these and other common behavioral and cognitive characteristics, such as poor impulse control, tangential speech, and difficulty in making transitions, may be caused by a lack of appropriate inhibition because of faulty brain connections.

COGNITIVE CHARACTERISTICS OF MALES

Each individual may exhibit many or only some of the characteristics expected from members of the group. As Pennington,

O'Connor, and Sudhalter remind us, "It is easy to forget that individuals with a given genetic syndrome are different in the vast majority of both their genes and their specific environmental experiences . . . It is unlikely that there will be a neuropsychological profile that is diagnostic of a genetic syndrome at the individual level" (1991, p. 176).

Information From Standardized Intelligence, Achievement, and Adaptive Behavior Testing

Intelligence test scores reported in the literature show a wide variation for both males and females. For males, whereas a majority of subjects whose scores are reported in the literature fall into the categories of moderate or severe mental retardation, many scores fall into the mild range, and a number have been reported in the average range and in the range between one and two standard deviations below the mean (Chudley, de von Flindt, & Hagerman, 1987; Curfs, Borghgraef, Schreppers-Tudink, & Fryns, 1989; Hagerman, Kemper, & Hudson, 1985; Madison, George, & Moeschler, 1986; Theobald, Hay, & Judge, 1987). Of these, most demonstrate learning disabilities.

Males with no evidence of mental retardation have often been discovered incidentally when entire families have been studied. This is a reminder that the persons with fragile X syndrome who have been available for study are those whose characteristics have brought them and/or their family members to attention for referral. So far, there have not been screenings of the general population to identify a fragile X syndrome sample (Pennington et al., 1991). Thus, there are people with fragile X syndrome whose characteristics have not caused them to be singled out or referred. When "typical characteristics" are described, or averages of test scores for a group of people with fragile X syndrome are stated, the more capable group of people with fragile X syndrome is obviously not included.

Score profiles on tests of intelligence have been studied to determine whether there are statistically significant patterns. The Wechsler Scales (Wechsler, 1974) have Verbal and Performance sections, each consisting of either five or six subtests. For males with fragile X syndrome, reports in the literature are not consistent in finding a significant difference between Verbal and Performance scores nor among subtest scores (Curfs et al., 1989). Apparently, the way that cognition is assessed by these scales does not assist either in identification of those who might have fragile X syndrome or in learning about their cognitive strengths and weaknesses.

More specific information about score profiles is given in two studies based on administration of the Kaufman Assessment Battery for Children (KABC) (Kaufman & Kaufman, 1983). This test reports a Mental Processing Composite score that is based on two scales: a Sequential Scale with items requiring a temporal or serial order of stimuli for solving problems, and a Simultaneous Scale that requires a gestalt-like, frequently spatial, integration of stimuli. Scores for the Achievement Scale, five subtests that assess acquisition of environmental information and performance on school-related tasks, are reported separately, and administration is at the discretion of the psychologist.

Kemper, Hagerman, and Altshul-Stark (1988), using the KABC (Kaufman & Kaufman, 1983), compared profiles of 20 boys who were cytogenetically positive for fragile X syndrome with 20 boys who were cytogenetically negative. The 40 boys ranged in age from 4 to 12 years, and all had KABC Mental Processing Composite scores ≥50. They found four significant profile differences between the performances of the boys with and without fragile X syndrome:

1. Simultaneous score higher than Sequential score (due to consistently higher performance on three of the five subtests);
2. Achievement score higher than the Mental Processing Composite score;
3. Matrix Analogies score higher than Spatial Memory score;
4. Arithmetic score less than the mean of the Achievement subtest scores.

Nineteen of the 20 boys with fragile X syndrome demonstrated at least three of these four profile patterns, while only 8 of the 20 boys without fragile X syndrome produced at least three of these patterns.

Dykens, Hodapp, and Leckman (1987) administered the KABC (Kaufman & Kaufman, 1983) to 14 boys and young men with fragile X syndrome. (The majority of their subjects were older than the upper standardization age of 12 1/2.) The resulting average scores support each of the four distinctive profile patterns reported by Kemper et al. (1988) for their subjects with fragile X syndrome.

Dykens, Hodapp, and Leckman (1989) reported test results on the Vineland Adaptive Behavior Scale (VABS) (Sparrow, Balla, & Cicchetti, 1984) for 27 males. Twelve of their subjects lived in a large state institution, ranged in age from 23 to 51 years, and had a mean IQ score of 22 (Stanford-Binet Form L-M). Fifteen lived at home or in small group homes, ranged in age from 3 to 28, and had a mean IQ score of 50 (range of 37 to 85) on the same test. The subjects represented a wide range of both age and measured intelligence test scores. Both groups demonstrated a significantly higher mean score in Daily Living Skills than in the domains of Communication and Socialization. Environmental effects may be hypothesized by the significantly higher Communication scores of those living in the community compared to those living in institutions, even though the former were a much younger group.

Bregman, Leckman, and Ort (1988) found scores on the VABS (Sparrow et al., 1984), including scores on the Socialization scale, to be significantly higher than intelligence test scores for 4 of 14 male subjects ranging in age from 3 to 27 years. One of their conclusions is that gaze aversion is caused by anxiety rather than autistic and social dysfunction.

Intelligence Test Score Changes With Age

Some researchers (Dykens, Hodapp, Ort, et al., 1989; Hagerman, et al., 1989; Lachiewicz, Gullion, Spiridigliozzi, & Aylsworth, 1987) have reported a decline in intelligence test scores for a majority, but not all, of their male subjects. (Decreases in intelligence test scores do not mean that children have lost skills or even that they have stopped increasing their skill repertoires. In order to receive a constant score on an intelligence test over time, a person must respond correctly to more questions as he gets older, usually to a ceiling of 16 years. If a person responds correctly either to the same number of questions or to only a few more questions while getting older, a decrease in score results.)

Examining data from these and other studies, Fisch et al. (1991) reported significant increases in scores for some subjects, even as others showed significant score decreases. They suggest that there may be at least two distinct clinical subtypes of males with fragile X syndrome, with one subtype demonstrating intellectual growth that continues at a stable rate, while the other demonstrates a slowing of intellectual growth after early or middle childhood (Fisch et al., in press).

We need to be very careful with interpretations of this information. The studies reported so far raise both methodological and theoretical questions. The research has been retrospective; that is, records of subjects have been used to determine earlier intelligence test scores. Thus, there has been no opportunity to compare subjects for *quality* of intervention. At best, only information about place of residence (home, group home, or institution) has been provided. Such factors as intensity of services, type and amount of occupational and speech and language therapy, and type of educational opportunities are not known.

There is both research evidence (Dykens et al., 1987) and a growing body of informal reports by teachers and therapists that many boys with fragile X syndrome demonstrate a higher level of skill on achievement tests and in the classoom than would be predicted by their intelligence test scores. This raises major research questions relative to intelligence test scores in general and reports of decline in intelligence test scores for males in particular:

1. What is the relationship between intelligence test scores, academic achievement, and adaptive behavior for children with fragile X syndrome?
2. Do academic achievement skills show patterns of change over time similar to or different from the changes in cognitive skills that are measured by intelligence tests?
3. What is the relationship between types and intensity of interventions and change in patterns of cognitive, academic achievement, and adaptive behavior skills?

To begin to answer these questions, children need to be followed from time of identification, with careful documentation of types and intensity of all services, including:

- Support to parents for managing and working with their children at home;
- Type and intensity of occupational and speech-language therapy;
- Educational opportunities;
- Determination of usefulness of medication and continual monitoring for effectiveness.

Cognitive Strengths and Weaknesses

Information about cognitive strengths and weaknesses comes from three sources: reports in the literature giving results from standardized intelligence and achievement testing, clinical reports based on observations by teachers and therapists, and reports based on parents' observations of their children. All three types of information will be employed in this section.

For discussion purposes, I have arbitrarily divided cognitive functioning into categories. The categories and the specific skills placed in them could be divided and grouped in many different ways. There is a great deal of interrelatedness among these categories, which is noted frequently in the information that follows. Specific suggestions are made, where possible, for restructuring or adapting tasks to decrease children's anxiety and frustration and increase learning. More general suggestions are given in a later section, Learning Style.

Memory

Intelligence tests measure short-term auditory memory by asking the subject to repeat series of numbers. The purest test of visual memory is a subtest on the Stanford-Binet, 4th Ed., that requires the reproduction of bead patterns by memory. People with fragile X syndrome perform more poorly on these types of tasks than on most other subtest tasks (Chudley et al., 1987; Curfs et al., 1989; Dykens et al., 1987; Kemper et al., 1988).

Because visual memory presents as a strength under many circumstances, poor performance on short-term auditory and visual memory subtests must involve factors other than the obvious suggestion of a weakness in this area. These alternative factors appear to be context and anxiety.

The matter of context is crucial for these children. There is a discrepancy between memory for contextual and for noncontextual material, particularly when the contextual material is of interest to the child. When children with fragile X syndrome are asked to remember something, whether presented auditorily or visually, that is not in context and not important to them (for example, a series of numbers on an intelligence test or a list of spelling words), their performance tends to be very poor. However, parents and teachers report that these same children often amaze them with their ability to remember events, often from years past, or to remember details about something of interest to themselves (for example, baseball statistics or information about certain types of automobiles).

Children with fragile X syndrome typically have a high level of anxiety, which also interferes with short-term memory tasks. When asked a question requiring production of remembered information, a child with fragile X syndrome is often unable to do so. However, this same child may spontaneously produce a great deal of remembered information, including information that could not be produced on specific request. The characteristic "block" when asked a direct question appears related to problems with word retrieval (see Chapter 5). Teachers and parents can help by giving time for the child to process a question and find the words to answer it. Use of "fill-ins" and indirect questions may also be effective.

Teaching students how to access information as needed is often a better use of instructional time than memorization drills. For example, rather than struggle to memorize his address, a student could learn, when asked his address, to retrieve from his wallet or pocket a card that has his address written on it. Require memorization of students with fragile X syndrome only when truly necessary. Most information that must be memorized is related to a context and, therefore, easier to learn. Reminders about the context can help the child produce the information.

Sequencing

A variety of commonly observed difficulties involve sequencing. Profile data from the KABC (Kaufman & Kaufman, 1983) show that tasks requiring sequencing are the most poorly performed (Dykens et al., 1987; Kemper et al., 1988).

Sequencing skills are required for a large number of classroom tasks. Following are examples of such tasks, responses of some boys with fragile X syndrome, and suggestions for assistance:

Task: Follow directions with more than one step.

Response: Student follows the first step of the direction, then stops.

Suggestion: Provide picture or written directions, one per page, and teach the student the process of following the direction on the first page, then turning it over, following the direction on the second page, and so on. This allows the specifics of the directions to change without changing the procedure of using the system.

Task: Follow a schedule.

Response: Student either (a) memorizes a typical schedule and is unable to deal with change or (b) tries to follow the schedule on the board but is unable to find the current place.

Suggestion: Provide an individual picture or written daily schedule, one activity per card, and teach the student the process of checking his schedule for the next activity, doing the activity, then turning the card over after the activity is completed. This allows the schedule to be changed without changing the procedure for following it. See McClennen (1991) for a detailed plan for teaching time management with picture schedules.

Task: Read using phonics.

Response: Student learns to match sounds and letters (especially consonants) but is unable to sequence sounds into words.

Suggestion: Teach a whole-word or word family approach to reading.

The difficulty with sequencing is probably related both to auditory memory, as expressed in tasks that require following a series of verbally presented directions, and to visuospatial skills, as required in tasks such as finding one's place in visual material. There may also be a relationship among difficulty in using phonics for reading, expressive language problems, and motor planning problems.

Visuospatial Skills

Children with fragile X syndrome behave in ways that suggest they have difficulty locating themselves in relation to the people and things in their environment. This difficulty may be a reason for their resistance to change in their environment and to transition from one activity to another. When one has worked very hard to figure out one's physical relationship to things in one's environment and has finally accomplished this task with a resultant feeling of safety and calm, a change in the environment or a move to a new environment causes the anxiety to begin all over again. This problem is certainly related to fragile X central nervous system dysfunction and to deficits in motor planning.

Reminders before transitions to make changes less abrupt help some children. Photographs of the next activity or environment, or of the way that the room will look after furniture is moved or another change is made, may help other children. Understanding why a child has difficulty with transitions and changes allows one to determine ways to help that child decrease or deal with the anxiety.

Two-dimensional space can also present visuospatial problems for children with fragile X syndrome. On the KABC (Kaufman & Kaufman, 1983) subtests Hand Movements (reproducing a series of hand movements) and Spatial Memory (remembering the locations of pictures in two-dimensional space), children with fragile X syndrome typically have lower scores than on other subtests (Dykens et al., 1987; Kemper et al., 1988). Tasks in two-dimensional space frequently have a sequencing component. The most obvious classroom activity for which this is relevant is handwriting, requiring both motor planning and cognitive sequencing skills.

Computers have made it possible for children for whom handwriting is terribly difficult to practice written expression. When all of one's energy goes into copying from the board or into trying to handwrite one's responses or ideas, there is no energy left for thinking and learning. Much less motor planning is required to hit a desired letter on a keyboard. A child with an educational goal of writing his name, rather than writing responses to questions to demonstrate learning, can learn to use name stamps at the proper place on the paper. Stamping is a visuospatial skill with a greatly reduced motor planning component. Some children, however, want to learn to write their own names when they see other children doing it and are often willing to work very hard at the task.

Math Skills

Children with fragile X syndrome, both boys and girls, demonstrate severe difficulties with mathematics skills compared to their skills in other areas (Dykens et al., 1987; Kemper et al., 1988). This is not surprising, because math performance requires two characteristics with which these children usually have particular difficulty: visuospatial skills and sequencing.

Beginning mathematics is built on the relationships of objects to each other, beginning with one-to-one correspondence. In order to solve problems, the student must perceive the relationships, decide on a course of action, then follow a step-by-step procedure to arrive at a solution. Children who do not have a particular difficulty with typical elementary school paper-and-pencil math instruction are those who can perceive relationships in their "mind's eye," understand the necessary steps, and follow them. However, many typical children need real objects in order to learn about the relationships of objects to each other and the manipulation of numbers to explain these relationships. This need for real objects is particularly true for children with fragile X syndrome.

An instructional program called PACE-Math™ was developed for children with this need (Grumblatt & McClennen, 1991). In the program, students learn procedures for manipulating real objects to solve real problems. Skills are carefully arranged according to difficulty, beginning with one-to-one correspondence and continuing through simple addition. The focus is on problem solving rather than on noncontextual memorizing. Money skills are included according to the degree of difficulty. Adaptations have been built in to encourage independence, such as the "dollar-more" method of paying for purchases to enable independent shopping for people who cannot dependably and accurately count change.

Speech and Language Skills

Speech and language characteristics are addressed in great detail in Chapter 5. Some of the more prominent problems in this area are late language development, poor intelligibility, perseverative speech, and difficulty answering direct questions because of problems with word retrieval and anxiety. A relative strength can be seen in vocabulary skills.

The relationship between language deficits and cognitive capabilities is not clear. There may be more than one cause for characteristics such as perseverative speech. For example, perseveration may be an attempt to "buy time" while trying to retrieve a word or a phrase. It may represent disordered thought, and it may be a manifestation of the child's cognitive level. Even the relative strength in vocabulary skills of children with fragile X syndrome needs further exploration. The skill may reflect understanding and remembrance of ideas in context, or it may reflect perseverative tendencies.

On the other hand, language provides an important coping skill for some students. A technique called "verbal rehearsal" consists of telling oneself what to do, then doing it. Children with fragile X syndrome can learn this technique through repeated practice: A parent, teacher, or therapist says, "Tell me how you are going to _____ ," waits for the child to explain, assists the child until he has stated it correctly, then encourages the child to follow his directions.

A new approach for identifying language and cognitive skills of people who are nonverbal or who have limited verbal skills is facilitated communication (Biklen, 1990). Its description is deceptively simple: supporting a person's arm and hand makes it possible for that person to direct a finger to his chosen spot on a keyboard. Pulling the person's hand back immediately following his choice of a letter prepares him to type the next letter. Calculator (1992) and McLean (1992) express their awareness that this technique is successful for a number of people and the need for research to explain the myriad of questions it raises.

I have found the following characteristics to indicate likelihood of success with facilitated communication: nonverbal or nonfunctionally verbal (e.g., echo what they hear rather than expressing themselves), demonstrate receptive language (e.g., "She understands an awfully lot"), have difficulty starting (follows some directions but not others that seem equally simple), have difficulty stopping (perseveration), have difficulty with fine motor skills (e.g., "He uses some signs but doesn't seem able to move his fingers into position for many others").

I have used this technique successfully with two nonverbal children with fragile X syndrome (in addition to 52 other children and adults with diagnoses of autism, cerebral palsy, or mental retardation). Both have IQ scores in the range of severe mental retardation, yet, with the technique of facilitated communication, have demonstrated literacy skills. This technique has also been used successfully at Ivymount School with one child with fragile X syndrome (in addition to others who have different diagnoses). As information and research on facilitated communication become available, children with fragile X syndrome with limited or no verbal skills should be considered as potential users of this technique for communication.

Organization

To be organized requires remembering, sequencing, and perceiving necessary objects in relation to each other. These are all typically areas of difficulty for children with fragile X syndrome. On the other hand, when an attempt is made to help the child organize by teaching a specific schedule for the day or directions for doing a task, and then a change in plans is required, the child cannot cope with the alteration.

As described earlier, it helps to teach students a procedure for using a schedule (so that the schedule can change without changing the procedure) and a procedure for following picture or written directions (so that the specifics of the directions can change without changing the procedure). By focusing on following the procedure, which doesn't change, some students can avoid the trauma they tend to experience from changes in the actual order of events. Picture or word lists with a procedure for using them can be used to teach students to gather materials for a project, for going home, or for getting ready for school.

Social Skills

Social interaction and communication are based on many skills that are especially difficult for children with fragile X syndrome. As a result, the youngsters often appear socially inappropriate. They seem to have few skills in identifying and responding to nonverbal cues. They say things that seem inappropriate to a current conversation. Sometimes, they avoid social interaction, appearing withdrawn or shy.

Social interaction skills can be taught. Peers with good social interaction skills are necessary for this process. After analyzing the skills typically used within an environment, provide opportunities for the child with fragile X syndrome to interact with socially adept children under structured circumstances where teaching can take place.

Visual Learning

Children with fragile X syndrome respond very well to visually presented information. The use of visual cues (for example, pictures, pointing, and demonstrating) paired with a verbal request often results in a successful response that does not occur from a verbal request alone. Parents often describe great variability in their children's ability or seeming willingness to respond to requests. Careful observation often shows that when the request is given in full sight of the child with a visual cue, the child is much more likely to respond correctly than when only the verbal request is made. Interestingly, sign language serves as a visual (and kinesthetic) cue for some children with fragile X syndrome as they learn to talk. Some preschoolers use sign language before they begin to speak.

On the KABC, (Kaufman & Kaufman, 1983) subjects with fragile X syndrome performed best on three subtests; Gestalt Closure, Matrix Analogies, and Faces & Places (Dykens et al., 1987; Kemper et al., 1988). On these subtests, sequencing is not necessary and all input is visually present, so the combination of sequencing and memory is not required. This is why it is helpful for children with fragile X syndrome to be given a sample or picture of a finished product before they begin work on it.

Imitation Skills

Modeling is the term used when an action is demonstrated for the student to imitate. Skill in imitation is a strength for children with fragile X syndrome. Their imitation ability builds on their strength in learning through visual cues and also on the children's positive interest in others. Visual learning and imitation skills enable children with fragile X syndrome to learn a wide variety of tasks that are necessary for independence in daily life and that are needed for many jobs.

Because children with fragile X syndrome have this strength and will imitate those around them, it is important to consider their role models. They will imitate the children who are their daily companions. Thus, if they are with children who demonstrate atypical or problem behaviors, they will imitate those behaviors. If they are with children who demonstrate appropriate behavior, they will imitate that.

Concrete vs. Abstract Thinking

Available evidence suggests that children with fragile X syndrome perform better when they are dealing with concrete rather than abstract tasks and materials. Cognitively, children must learn to cope with the concrete world before they can learn to respond to abstractions. Given the challenge of learning to locate themselves in space, the positive response of children with fragile X syndrome to visual learning and imitative modeling, combined with their difficulty in verbal expression, sequencing, and organization, their need for the concrete is not surprising.

Many people with fragile X syndrome demonstrate a sense of humor. Parents often report that their children derive a great deal of enjoyment from slapstick humor, which is usually literal and concrete.

Skills for Solving Life's Little Problems

Finally, Dever (1988) points out that we often teach people as if each day will progress perfectly. In reality, life is full of glitches— the little things that go wrong daily that must be dealt with. Shoelaces break. Your favorite cereal has run out. Interventions need to be developed to teach people with fragile X syndrome how to deal with the glitches of life so they will not constantly be overwhelmed by them. Interventions include learning to buy an extra before the product you use has run out, substitution and replacement (for example, selecting a different pair of shoes when the laces have broken on one's favorites, then buying new shoelaces), and calling the relevant person when a bus is missed resulting in late arrival.

COGNITIVE CHARACTERISTICS OF FEMALES

Fewer studies have been done addressing females than those addressing males. Of these few studies, most have focused on adults or a mixed group of adults and children. Among women studied who are obligate carriers (they have given birth to sons with fragile X syndrome), signifcant differences have been described between groups of fra(X)-negative and fra(X)-positive women (Brainard, Schreiner, & Hagerman, 1991; Prouty et al., 1988). The former appear cognitively unimpaired, but scores of the latter group are concentrated in the low-average to mild retardation ranges. Among all obligate carriers with IQ scores in the average range, there is a significantly greater number with specific learning disabilities than among a matched group without fragile X syndrome.

While no consistent difference has been found between scores on the Verbal and Performance scales of the Wechsler Adult Intelligence Scale-Revised (WAIS-R) (Wechsler, 1981) for either group, several studies have found subtest differences for fra(X)-positive women and girls. On the Wechsler scales, fra(X)-positive women, including those with IQ scores in the average range, have consistently shown weaknesses on the subscales of arithmetic, digit span, and block design (Pennington et al., 1991). On the Stanford-Binet, 4th Ed. (Thorndike, Hagen, & Sattler, 1985), Freund and Reiss (1989) and Freund (1991) descibe a pattern of performance for nonretarded girls who are fra(X)-positive that suggests a strength in processing and remembering information in verbal form and a deficit in remembering and processing information that is not easily labeled. This information from intelligence test subtest profiles suggests a milder version of some of the difficulties experienced by males: remembering noncontextual information (especially if it is based on abstractions that are not easily labeled), visuospatial tasks, and arithmetic.

Another area of difficulty for females with fragile X syndrome is usually described as a social difficulty: shyness, being withdrawn, appearing uncomfortable around others, and having limited friendships and peer relationships (Freund, 1991). These behaviors may be based on cognitive problems in identifying and responding to the social cues and nonverbal behavior of others and can result in behaviors that look socially maladaptive. If this is the case, efforts must be made to teach the skills necessary to increase positive social interaction.

Although group patterns for females can be identified, many individuals do not demonstrate them. Thus, each girl must be addressed as a individual, but it is important to be watchful for the specific areas of deficit that have been identified in order to provide useful interventions. The use of verbal mediation strategies, such as verbal rehearsal and learning to translate visual information into verbal form, particularly fits the cognitive pattern that is emerging for girls with fragile X syndrome.

The literature does not address cognitive characteristics for girls and women with fragile X syndrome who have mental retardation. Careful individual assessment should provide useful information for planning intervention.

ASSESSMENT

Assessment should be approached as an opportunity to learn about the type and intensity of intervention required, rather than as a measurement of the degree of deficit. When a child scores at or above the average range on a standardized test of intelligence and is performing commensurately in school, the assumption is either that there is no need for special interventions or that interventions already in place are adequate. When a child's score is in or near the range identified for mental retardation, the assumption is that without intervention the child will fail in school. We will be most helpful to children by responding to low scores with the recognition that the child is very vulnerable and needs intensive intervention, rather than using low scores as an excuse to minimize intervention.

Psychologists engaged in intelligence testing and others performing formal speech and language or educational achievement assessment want to assess cognitive ability as accurately as possible in spite of the behavioral, language, and attentional characteristics typical of children with fragile X syndrome. Following are considerations for achieving this goal.

Formal Assessment

Experienced assessors will already be employing many of the suggestions to be described, in addition to others not mentioned here. However, this list can serve as a reminder when preparations are made to assess a student with fragile X syndrome.

Familiarity

Children with fragile X syndrome find it very difficult to orient to their surroundings. It is not atypical for the person responsible for formal assessment, who is largely or totally unfamiliar to a child, to take this child to an unfamiliar office or clinic for testing. This results in very high anxiety based on change in routine, unfamiliarity with the assessor, and difficulty orienting to a new place. No one does well in a situation where anxiety is very high, and children with fragile X syndrome demonstrate much higher anxiety than others.

To avoid this problem, the child must have time before beginning formal testing to become familiar with the assessor and with the place where testing will occur. This may require a great deal of time and more than one visit. These visits can be profitably used for observation and planned informal testing utilizing game-like and indirect requests.

Time of Day

Most children perform best in the morning. All children have predictable times of the day when they are "at their best." This is even more true for children with fragile X syndrome than for typical children, and it is especially true for children on medication related to hyperactivity or anxiety. It is crucial to understand the child's biological schedule and to accommodate to it. Test at a time when the student is most attentive and responsive.

Length of Sessions

Children with fragile X syndrome perform better when tested during short sessions over many days rather than one or two long sessions. In addition, this allows the assessor to observe possible differences in behavior and responses on different days. Also, through discussions with parents and teachers, the assessor can determine more about the relationship between timing of medication, general affect, and response to the assessment situation.

Calming

Using calming techniques identified by the child's occupational therapist will assist the child to focus on assessment tasks. Depending on the child, calming techniques might be performed before testing and even during testing. These techniques could be learned by the psychologist or other assessor or could be perfomed by a person who regularly uses them with the child.

Seating

Often, children with fragile X syndrome are more comfortable and can perform better when they can sit in a beanbag chair, on the floor, or in some other previously identified way. While they must learn to sit in a typical school chair most of the time, it is important to reduce stress as much as possible during testing.

Reinforcement

Tangible reinforcers for *attempts* to respond can help some children. (Do not require correct response; do not reinforce no response or disruptive responses.) Use a very concrete system, such as boxes that can be checked or starred. When a set of checks (on a card, line, or page) is completed, deliver the reinforcer. When the next set of checks is completed, give the next reinforcer, and so on. The number of attempted responses required for reinforcement depends on both the age and degree of hyperactivity of the child.

Refocusing

It is not uncommon for children with fragile X syndrome to shift focus to some other subject or to make comments that may appear to have no meaning in the current context. This can even happen in the middle of a task. In this event, refocus the student's attention on the task at hand. In a gentle voice, repeat the direction. Point to the materials with which the student should be working or at which the student should be looking. It is usually best not to mention the irrelevant comments, but only to call attention to the task.

Learning from Mistakes

A great deal of information can be learned from careful attention to the exact nature of incorrect responses. Although it doesn't affect scoring, the following information will be of great assistance in understanding the child's cognitive style:

- Are incorrect responses reasonable or totally off the mark?
- Was the child "saying anything" in an attempt to be compliant although not paying attention, or was he appearing to be attending and trying, yet still responding incorrectly?
- Do incorrect responses appear to be caused by difficulties in focusing, which can be seen in inconsistent patterns of correct responses within subtests, or are easy items correct, followed by increasingly incorrect responses as items become more difficult for the child?

Informal Assessment

Adaptations of Test Items

Children with fragile X syndrome often perform better when the format of test materials is changed. For example, adapt tests that use pictures, such as parts of the Woodcock-Johnson Psychoeducational Battery (Woodcock, 1978) by having only one picture per page. Children have performed better when the pictures are laid out in a straight line rather than in a square configuration, such as on the Peabody Picture Vocabulary Test-R (Dunn & Dunn, 1981). Compare a child's scores with and without this adaptation. If a child performs better using a specific format, there are implications for presentation of schoolwork.

Direct vs. Indirect Assessment

When asked directly, many of these children cannot always perform skills that they can and do perform when encouraged indirectly or when they themselves initiate performance of the skill. For example, a child who could not calculate an arithmetic problem when asked could look at another student's paper and tell whether that student was doing each problem correctly or not. Indirect assessment enables evaluation of children's cognitive abilities through game-like situations and through opportunities to "catch" youngsters doing skills when there is no pressure.

Interpretation of Test Results

Current evidence supports higher academic achievement for boys with fragile X syndrome than would have been predicted by their intelligence test scores alone. Studies described earlier in this chapter found that children with fragile X syndrome scored significantly higher on the Achievement Scale than on the Mental Processing Composite of the KABC, (Kaufman & Kaufman, 1983) while the control group used in one of the studies scored about the same on both scales. Teachers have reported informally and I have observed a number of boys with fragile X syndrome who demonstrate academic skills in school much higher than those that might be anticipated, based on intelligence test scores.

It is plausible that the characteristic behaviors of hyperactivity, lack of attention, and impulsivity, coupled with the need for context related to their experiences that is observed in boys with fragile X syndrome, interfere with their performance on intelligence tests. This suggests that the children's intelligence test scores should be considered as a statement of minimum performance, not as a statement of potential, or even as typical of current ability. The focus should be on what can be learned from the testing situation, both formally and informally, rather than on scores. With the goal of identifying the most helpful approaches to intervention, assessors can learn a great deal from observation, from analysis of both correct and incorrect responses, and from analysis of their own behaviors that supported or impeded a student's efforts.

Instruments for Intelligence Testing

For children between the ages of 2 1/2 and 12 1/2, the Kaufman Assessment Battery for Children (KABC) (Kaufman & Kaufman, 1983) is recommended. There are three reasons. First, this test includes many nonverbal scales, and those scales that do require verbal responses usually require only single word responses. This allows separation of the speech and language problems from cognitive assessment as measured by an intelligence test. Secondly, the KABC includes an Achievement Scale in addition to the Mental Processing Composite Scale. Because scales were standardized together, direct comparison of scores is possible. Third, and perhaps most important, the KABC was standardized with opportunities to "teach the test." The psychologist often experiences frustration from the belief that a particular child could respond better if it were possible to teach the child how to do a particular type of test item. Built into the test (and its standardization) are instructions for teaching the child how to perform the items for any scale where the child does not demonstrate correct responses on sample or beginning items for that scale. Children with fragile X syndrome perform better as familiarity with the task increases.

Infants and toddlers are best assessed by the Bayley Scale of Infant Development (Bayley, 1969) (2 months to 3 years). This test has separate motor and mental scales and assesses a wide variety of skills. For teenagers and adults, the Stanford-Binet, 4th Ed., (Terman & Merrill, 1972) and the Wechsler Intelligence Scale for Children-Revised (Wechsler, 1974) or Wechsler Adult Intelligence Scale-Revised (Wechsler, 1981) assesses only hearing vocabulary through picture selection and is not considered a valid intelligence test. At this writing, a distinctive profile for boys with fragile X sydrome has been reported only for the KABC.

Tests to Avoid

The Leiter, often used with nonverbal children, is not a good choice for children with fragile X syndrome because of the heavy reliance on visuospatial ability, which tends to be a weakness for these children. The items on the Stanford-Binet Form L-M (Terman & Merrill, 1972) are 50 years old. The most recent restandardization was done in 1972—20 years ago. There is a new Stanford-Binet. It is time to lay the old one to rest.

LEARNING STYLE

Providing an environment for learning requires attention to behavioral as well as cognitive characteristics. The cause-and-effect relationships between cognitive and behavioral characteristics are being researched. As these relationships are identified, we will be more effective in implementing helpful interventions. In the meantime, therapists and teachers must make "educated guesses" based on current knowledge and observations.

Common behaviors, such as hand biting and flapping, gaze avoidance, tactile defensiveness, and perseverative speech, show a marked increase at times of high anxiety. At such times, learning is not likely to take place. The child needs to lower his anxiety, whether through calming, removing himself from sensory overload, or some other means. Sometimes, such behaviors tell teachers or therapists that the adult's requests are inappropriate and need to be modified.

The environment should be as comfortable for the child with fragile X syndrome as possible. Examples are:

- Fidgeting, as long as it doesn't disturb others, certainly should be permissible.
- Opportunities to move around should be more frequent than for others of the same age.
- There should be much more doing than listening activities.
- Headphones with calming music help block out auditory overload for some children.
- When a student demonstrates gaze aversion, allow him to sit where he doesn't have to face the teacher all the time.
- One child is reported to participate in group time by sitting in a rocking chair with a book.

Develop opportunities for the child to leave the room in a nonpunitive way. One teacher has arranged with a colleague to accept an envelope from her student with fragile X syndrome at any time. When the student begins to show signs of anxiety and agitation, his teacher asks him to please take a message to Ms. Davis. The teaching assistant goes with him. When they return a few moments later, he is ready to work again. He may have been calmed by the movement, the focus on a task he enjoys, or removing himself from the hustle and bustle of his classroom.

Teaching must take advantage of the child's strengths and assist the child in coping with his deficits. We must use what we know about cognitive strengths of children with fragile X syndrome in planning instruction.

Context is very important. Just as speech and language skills must be taught in the context of purposeful communication, so must the academic skills of reading (or use of picture lists and directions), arithmetic, and written expression be taught in the context of purposeful accomplishment of tasks that require the skills.

Otherwise, the material will be learned as rote exercises rather than as problem solving skills.

We can help these children organize by teaching them procedures that can be adapted to a wide variety of purposes. The child who has learned to follow pictured or written directions will be able to perform a large number of tasks that he could never do by memory.

These children often demonstrate very specific (and sometimes narrow) interests. Whenever possible, that interest should be used in the service of instruction. For example, if the student is interested in rocks, rocks can be used as the basis for instruction and assignments in reading (read about rocks), arithmetic (match, count, or add rocks), written expression, and, of course, science.

Children with fragile X syndrome often have a good sense of humor. Gentle humor can make any activity more interesting. Therapists and teachers have found humor particularly useful in role play to increase communication and social skills.

While these children often begin talking later than usual and may exhibit unusual speech patterns, once they have learned to talk, they may use speech to help them cope and problem solve. For example, some use the technique of verbal rehearsal (described earlier) in which they first tell themselves what to do, then do it. Teach this skill if the student has not learned it and suggest and encourage its use once it is learned.

Visual learning is a strength. Visual cues can be given in a wide variety of ways. A colored dot or arrow designates the place to begin on the left side of the worksheet. A child's photograph or name identifies his locker. When a visual cue accompanies spoken requests or instructions, the student is much more likely to understand and respond correctly. Use the child's response to the visual gestalt. Whenever possible, help the child see the goal.

School Placement

In many school districts and programs, there is an assumption that children with disabilities should be placed in classes with children whose intelligence test scores are similar to their own. In reality, there has long been evidence that intelligence test scores are likely to misrepresent ability to learn. Fifty years ago, Inhelder (1968 translation of 1943 French publication) examined the development of reasoning. Her subjects included both children and adults, ages 7 to 52, with Binet IQ scores ranging from 42 to 104. Each subject was assessed individually on a variety of conservation tasks using the Piagetian clinical method. She found that for many subjects there was no relationship between performance on cognitive tasks and their intelligence test scores. In some instances, a high degree of verbal facility, often coupled with good memory, produced relatively high intelligence test scores that masked reasoning only developed to the intuitional stage of the preoperational period. In other instances, limited verbal facility, often coupled with poor memory, poor school performance, and limited attention resulted in underassessment of reasoning ability.

As described earlier, the characteristic behaviors of hyperactivity, lack of attention, and impulsivity, coupled with the need for context related to their experiences that is observed in children with fragile X syndrome, interfere with their performance on intelligence tests. My experience with children with fragile X syndrome has been that their intelligence test scores, including those based on my own administration, underrepresent their abiilty to learn. Scores suggesting lower ability levels than actually exist can result in school placement with children whose cognitive skills are less advanced than the child with fragile X syndrome and in lowered expectations on the part of the teacher. The lack of cognitive challenge can result in boredom, which exacerbates the behavioral and attentional characteristics, and the lack of a cognitively equal or superior peer group does not provide good problem solving or language models, which further exacerbates the cognitive and language deficits.

The discrepancy between performance on intelligence tests and much higher performance when appropriate interventions are provided in a classroom setting must be taken into consideration when school placements are being decided. There is evidence that a large majority of children with disabilities learn additional skills when they are included in a general education class with other students of their chronological age, but with educational goals appropriate for them that may be different from those of their classmates. Also necessary are the supports and services to make the arrangement work to everyone's benefit (Ford et al., 1989; Schnorr, Ford, Davern, Park-Lee, & Meyer,1989; Stainback, Stainback, & Forest, 1989).

Being educated with typical children of the same age is particularly appropriate for children with fragile X syndrome. These children are very sociable in spite of their specific difficulties in learning social skills. They are much more likely to learn good social skills from typical peers. Children with fragile X syndrome are visual learners. They learn best by watching what others do. Like all children, they learn from peers at least as much, if not more, than they learn from adults. Being part of a regular classroom provides continuous opportunity to learn by modeling from peers. It is not unusual for children with fragile X syndrome to demonstrate many more cognitive and social skills after they have joined a regular class (Lancaster, 1991). Being with typical peers can also work well for preschool children—again, as long as necessary supports and services are provided (Buysse & Bailey, 1991).

Children with fragile X syndrome have been described as hyperactive, frustrated, withdrawn, distractible, self-injurious, and so on. It is important to remember that these are not character deficits of children with fragile X syndrome, but rather the result of their cognitive and neurological characteristics. As we identify these children, identify their individual strengths and deficits, and plan interventions that help them cope with finding the tasks of life very hard, they will thank us with behavior that will make their and our lives more pleasant. They are loving children and want to please. We must find and give them the tools.

REFERENCES

Bayley, N. (1969). *Bayley Scales of Infant Development.* New York: Psychological Corporation.

Biklen, D. (1990). Communication unbound: Autism and praxis. *Harvard Educational Review, 60,* 291-314.

Brainard, S.S., Schreiner, R.A., & Hagerman, R.J. (1991). Cognitive profiles of the adult carrier fra(X) female. *American Journal of Medical Genetics, 38,* 505-508.

Bregman, J. D., Leckman, J. F., & Ort, S. I. (1988). Fragile X syndrome: Genetic predisposition to psychopathology. *Journal of Autism and Developmental Disorders, 17,* 469-486.

Buysse, V., & Bailey, D. (1991, Holiday Issue). Mainstreaming young children with disabilities: What have we learned? *Fragile X Southeast News,* 4-5.

Calculator, S. (1992). Perhaps the emperor has clothes after all: A response to Biklen. *American Journal of Speech-Language Pathology, 1,* 18-20.

Chudley, A. E., de von Flindt, R., & Hagerman, R. J. (1987). Invited editorial comment: Cognitive variability in the fragile X syndrome. *American Journal of Medical Genetics, 28,* 13-15.

Curfs, L. M. G., Borghgraef, M., Wiegers, A., Schreppers-Tudink, G. A. J., & Fryns, J. P. (1989). Strengths and weaknesses in the cognitive profile of fragile X patients. *Clinical Genetics, 36,* 405-410.

Dever, R. B. (1988). *Community living skills: A taxonomy.* (Monographs No. 10) Washington, DC: American Association on Mental Retardation.

Dunn, L., & Dunn, L. (1981). *Peabody Picture Vocabulary Test-Revised.* Circle Pines, American Guidance Service.

Dykens, E. M., Hodapp, R. M., & Leckman, J. F. (1989). Adaptive and maladaptive functioning of institutionalized and noninstitutionalized fragile X males. *Journal of American Academic Child and Adolescent Psychiatry,* *28,* 427-430.

Dykens, E.M., Hodapp, R.M., & Leckman, J.F. (1987). Strengths and weaknesses in the intellectual functioning of males with fragile X syndrome. *American Journal of Mental Deficiency, 92,* 234-236.

Dykens, S. M. , Hodapp, R. M., Ort, S., Finucane, B., Shapiro, L. R., & Leckman, J. F. (1989). The trajectory of cognitive development in males with fragile X syndrome. *Journal of American Academy of Child and Adolescent Psychiatry, 28,* 422-426.

Fisch, G. S., Arinami, T., Froster-Iskenius, U., Fryns, J., Curfs, L.M., Borghgraef, M., Howard-Peebles, P. N., Schwartz, C. E., Simensen, R. J., & Shapiro, L. R. (1991). Relationship between age and IQ among fragile X males: A multicenter study. *American Journal of Medical Genetics, 38,* 481-487.

Fisch, G. S., Shapiro, L. R., Simensen, R., Schwartz, C. E., Fryns, J. P., Borghgraef, M., Curfs, L. M., Howard-Peebles, P. N., Arinami, T., & Mavrou, A. (in press). Longitudinal changes in IQ among fragile X males: Clinical evidence of more than one mutation? *American Journal of Medical Genetics.*

Ford, A., Schnorr, R., Meyer, L., Davern, L., Black, J., & Dempsey, P. (1989). The Syracuse community-referenced curriculum guide for students with moderate and severe disabilities. Baltimore: Brookes.

Freund, L., & Reiss, A. L. (1989, July). Cognitive profile comparisons of fragile X males and females. Presented at the Fourth International Workshop on Fragile X Syndrome and X-linked Mental Retardation, New York.

Freund, L. (1991, Summer/Fall). Clinical research updates on the female with fragile X. *Fragile X Southeast News,* 4-6.

Grumblatt, L., & McClennen, S. (1991). Math is more than counting. In S. McClennen, *Cognitive skills for community living: Teaching students with moderate to severe disabilities.* Austin, TX: PRO-ED.

Hagerman, R. J. (1991). Physical and behavioral phenotype. In R. J. Hagerman & A. C. Silverman (Eds.), *Fragile X syndrome: Diagnosis, treatment, and research* (pp. 3-68). Baltimore: Johns Hopkins University Press.

Hagerman, R. J., Kemper, M., & Hudson, M. (1985). Learning disabilities and attentional problems in boys with the fragile X syndrome. *American Journal of Diseases in Children, 139,* 674-678.

Hagerman, R. J., Schreiner, R. A., Kemper, M. B., Wittenberger, M. D., Zahn, B., & Habicht, K. (1989). Longitudinal IQ changes in fragile X males. *American Journal of Medical Genetics, 33,* 513-518.

Inhelder, B. (1968). *The diagnosis of reasoning in the mentally retarded.* New York: The John Day Co.

Kaufman, A. S., & Kaufman, N. L. (1983). *Kaufman assessment battery for children.* Circle Pines, MN: American Guidance Services.

Kemper, L.B., Hagerman, R.J., & Altshul-Stark, D. (1988). Cognitive profiles of boys with fragile X syndrome. *American Journal of Medical Genetics, 30,* 191-200.

Lachiewicz, A. M., Gullion, C. M., Spiridigliozzi, G. A., & Aylsworth, A. S. (1987). Declining IQs of young males with the fragile X syndrome. *American Journal of Mental Retardation, 92,* 272-278.

Lancaster, J. (1991, Spring/Summer). Integration: A positive view. *The National Fragile X Foundation Newsletter*, 4-6.

Madison, L., George, C., & Moeschler, J. (1986). Cognitive functioning in the fragile X syndrome: A study of intellectual, memory and communication skills. *Journal of Mental Deficiency Research, 30*, 129-148.

McLean, J. (1992). Facilitated communication: Some thoughts on Biklen's and Calculator's interaction. *American Journal of Speech-Language Pathology, 1*, 25- 27.

Pennington, B. F., O'Connor, R. A., & Sudhalter, V. (1991). Toward a neuropsychology of fragile X syndrome. In R. J. Hagerman & A. C. Silverman (Eds.), *Fragile X syndrome: Diagnosis, treatment, and research* (pp. 173-201). Baltimore: Johns Hopkins University Press.

Prouty, L.A., Roger, R.C., Stevenson, R.E., Dean, J.H., Palmer, K.K., Simenson, R.J., Coston, G.N., & Schwartz, C.E. (1988). Fragile X syndrome: Growth, development, and intellectual function. *American Journal of Medical Genetics, 30*, 123-142.

Sparrow, S., Balla, D., & Cicchetti, D. (1984). Vineland scales of adaptive behavior, survey form manual. Circle Pines, MN: American Guidance Service.

Schnorr, R., Ford, A., Davern, L., Park-Lee, S., & Meyer, L. (1989). *The Syracuse curriculum revision manual.* Baltimore: Brookes.

Stainback, S., Stainback, W., & Forest, M. (1989). *Educating all students in the mainstream of regular education.* Baltimore: Brookes.

Theobald, T., Hay, D., & Judge, C. (1987). Individual variation and specific cognitive deficits in fragile X syndrome. *American Journal of Medical Genetics, 28*, 1-11.

Thorndike, R.L., Hagen, E.P., & Sattler, J.M. (1985). *Stanford-Binet Intelligence Scale, 4th Ed.* Chicago: Riverside.

Wechsler, D. (1974). *Wechsler Intelligence Scale for Children-Revised.* New York: Psychological Corporation.

Wechsler, D. (1981). *Wechsler Adult Intelligence Scale-Revised.* New York: Psychological Corporation.

Woodcock, R. (1978). *Woodcock-Johnson Psychoeducational Battery.* Hingham, Teaching Resources Corporation.

4

MOTOR AND SENSORY CHARACTERISTICS OF FRAGILE X

The diagnosis of fragile X syndrome is accompanied by well-documented and fairly stereotypical delays in gross and fine motor development, difficulties in effectively processing information from the basic sensory systems, and impairments in behavior, organizational skills, and attentional abilities that are related to deficits in sensory integration. Ayres (1973) suggests that adequate early motor and sensory development leads to a well-functioning, mature organism able to perceive, integrate, and react purposefully to his environment. Sensory integration is a term Ayres uses to describe the organization of sensations to be interpreted and used by the nervous system. The organization results in smooth, automatic, responsive movement. Children with fragile X often demonstrate behavioral reactions that are triggered by an overload or miscommunication of sensory input. Many use a variety of sensory-based behaviors to enhance input to their basic sensory systems in an attempt to make sense of their environment.

GROSS MOTOR

Delays in both gross and fine motor development are seen in persons with fragile X. Most often, motor skill levels are commensurate with cognitive levels. These delays in the acquisition of skills are not as significant as the qualitative deficits seen in normal movement patterns. For example, in studies reported by Levitas, Braden, Van Norman, Hagerman, and McBogg (1983), the onset of walking is almost always by age 2. The quality of the gait, however, is often affected by two primary motor characteristics of fragile X: joint laxity, which is seen as a result of an associated connective-tissue disorder, and hypotonia (low muscle tone). The joint laxity results in less proximal stability at the joints; therefore, movement occurs from a base less stable than ideal. Hypotonia, or low muscle tone, can also have an effect on the acquisition of motor milestones and quality movement. In addition, low muscle tone and joint laxity put an individual at risk for foot and spinal malalignments. According to Davids, Hagerman, and Eilkert (1990), 75% of males with fragile X have flat feet and many walk with a duck-like gait, characterized by a collapsed medial arch with pronation of the fore part of the foot and valgus angulation of the hind part of the foot. Individuals with fragile X have a greater incidence of scoliosis than the general population. Balance is the most frequently affected component within the motor area. Individuals with fragile X have difficulty with abilities requiring balance, such as standing on one foot, hopping, jumping, and skilled movement. This impairment in balance may be due in part to the low tone and joint laxity, but is also felt to be caused by a sensory integration problem relating to the vestibular system known as gravitational insecurity.

FINE MOTOR

Fine motor skills can also be delayed in children with fragile X syndrome. Again, it is the hypotonia and joint laxity that contribute to delays in the use of the hands for precision movement. Both lack of strength and the delay in the development of precision grasp can affect the quality of fine motor skills. Laxity of the ligaments in wrists, hands and fingers can cause joint instability, so problems may be seen in grasping and with such resistive fine motor activities as snapping and buttoning closures. Fine motor development is directly related to the level of cognitive functioning. The tactile hypersensitivity demonstrated by many children with fragile X can also have a negative effect on fine motor development. For example, the child who cannot tolerate the feel of a writing tool in his hand will exhibit poor or absent handwriting. The ocular-motor deficits and visual-spatial implications cited later in this chapter will have an effect on the development of visual and perceptual motor skills. The effects of joint laxity, tactile hypersensitivity, and delays caused by cognitive limitations contribute to impaired fine motor functioning.

TACTILE SYSTEM

The tactile system is human beings' oldest and largest sensory system, with receptors covering our bodies. Tactile receptors are located in the skin. The proprioceptive system, with receptors located in joints and tendons, is closely associated with the tactile system. Together these two sensory systems combine to form what is called somatosensory processing. There is often close interaction between touch and joint and body movement: it can be difficult to separate the influence of these two sensory systems. Both systems develop early in utero and are thought to play a primary role in early development. They serve as foundations for social, emotional, and, possibly, academic development.

The tactile system serves two functions: protection and discrimination. It is a fine-tuned system that must maintain a balance between these two functions for an individual to be able to successfully integrate and use information. The protective system helps a person keep safe by sensing danger from touch, pressure, pain, and temperature. If you have mistakenly touched a hot stove, you experienced this protective channel at work as you quickly withdrew your hand. The discriminatory function enables us to feel and recognize objects placed in our hands without the use of vision. It is this system that allows us to reach into our pockets and identify a dime in a pocketful of change.

The two identified disorders of the tactile system, tactile defensiveness and poor tactile discrimination, are felt to be central processing disorders. Stimuli enter through the skin, are received by a peripheral receptor, and are carried to the spinal cord by afferent fibers. They are then transmitted to the brain for processing by either the dorsal column medial lemniscal system for tactile, vibratory, touch-pressure, and proprioceptive information or the anterolateral system for pain, crude touch, and temperature.

Tactile Defensiveness

Eighty percent (Levitas et al.,1983) of males with fragile X are reported to have some degree of tactile defensiveness or aversion to being touched or to touching. This occurs because the protective function of the tactile system overrides the discrimination portion, causing seemingly harmless touch to be perceived by the individual as dangerous or noxious. Tactile defensiveness is hypothesized to be a disorder in the modulation or regulation of tactile sensory input (Clark, Mailloux, & Parham, 1989). The following chart by Royeen (1985) describes the behaviors of tactile defensiveness as follows:

1. Avoidance of touch:
   a. Avoidance of certain styles or textures (e.g., scratchy or rough) of clothing or, conversely, an unusual preference for certain styles or textures of clothing (e.g., soft materials, long pants, or sleeves);
   b. Preference for standing at the end of a line to avoid contact with other children
   c. Tendency to pull away from anticipated touch or from interactions involving touch, including avoidance of touch to face;
   d. Avoidance of play activities that involve body contact (can be manifested by a tendency to prefer solitary play).

2. Aversive responses to non-noxious touch:
   a. Aversion or struggle when picked up, hugged, or cuddled;
   b. Aversion to certain daily living tasks, including baths, cutting of fingernails, haircuts, and face washing;
   c. Aversion to dental care;
   d. Aversion to art materials, including avoidance of finger paints, paste, or sand.

3. Atypical affective responses to non-noxious tactile stimuli:
   a. Responding with aggression to light touch to arms, face, or legs;
   b. Increased stress in response to being physically close to people;
   c. Objection, withdrawal, or negative responses to touch contact, including that encountered in the context of intimate relationships.

Tactile defensiveness has been closely correlated with emotional difficulties, attention deficit, and hyperactivity. Recently it has been speculated that tactile defensiveness can predispose an individual to irregular emotional tone, lability, extreme need for personal space, and a disruption in personal intimate relationships (Wilbarger & Royeen, 1987).

Poor Tactile Discrimination

Tactile discrimination is the ability to perceive what you feel. Deficits in tactile perception can impair a person's ability to feel where or how many times he is touched and to recognize the shape of an object through touch (stereognosis). These deficits can interfere with the efficiency of how an individual tactually explores and handles items and may also be connected to impaired awareness of self (body scheme). Deficits in tactile discrimination are varied in individuals with fragile X, but fine motor delays and impaired awareness of self are commonly seen in the fragile X population.

VESTIBULAR SYSTEM

The vestibular system responds to position and movement of the head and to the effects of gravity on the body. The receptors for this system are located in the inner ear in the semicircular canals, the utricle, and the saccule. The effects of the vestibular system are closely related to the visual system and the proprioceptive system. Until recently, literature always separated the vestibular and proprioceptive systems; currently, they are being combined and referred to as the vestibular-proprioceptive system (Fisher, 1991). Both systems respond to movement, with the vestibular system responding to the sensation of movement of and to the body, and proprioception responding to the movement within the body. For the purpose of discussing the characteristics of fragile X, this chapter will deal with the systems separately. The three major functions of the vestibular system are (Fisher, 1991):

1. Awareness of body position, movement position, and movement in space;
2. Postural tone and equilibrium;
3. Stabilization of eyes in space during head movement (compensatory eye movement).

Problems seen when there is inadequate processing in the vestibular system are on a continuum, ranging from underreactivity to hyperactivity. The first problem we will discuss is under-registration or under-perception of vestibular input. In this case, an individual is not getting enough information to his brain from his vestibular receptors. This is the case with the child who does not develop adequate postural mechanisms in order to have an active upright posture against gravity. He has difficulty with the development and refinement of coordination, both in gross and fine motor skills. He also may lack the ability to smoothly coordinate and organize his eye movements. Another difficulty for this child is maintaining a calm and alert state. This child is typically low-tone and has difficulty maintaining an upright standing or sitting posture. This child may have difficulty sitting still; he needs the constant movement of moving around in his seat and wandering about the classroom. The excessive movement of these children is an attempt to feed information into their vestibular receptors so their brain can respond with better posture and a calm and alert state. They also need to move because their balance and equilibrium responses are so inadequate that they have poor control of their body when they are still and actually do better when they are in motion. The opposite end of that vestibular continuum is the individual who misperceives or receives too much input from gravity or movement. This results in a situation where the individual is threatened and very fearful of sometimes the slightest movement or balance challenge. This is referred to as gravitational or postural insecurity. This disorder is also on a continuum and can range from fear of heights to the inability to step off a curb without feeling that they are threatened and may fall. This fear is very real and, just as with tactile hypersensitivity, even the thought of movement challenge can evoke a flight-or-fright phenomenon. As you can imagine, this fear causes a major disruption in the child's inner drive. He is afraid to move, but desperately wants to run, climb, play, and enjoy. To control this excessive reaction to input, this child often holds his head as still as possible, so he looks quite rigid as he moves about. In addition to a rigid body, he also may develop a rigid, controlling, or inflexible personality that may be his attempt to manipulate people and objects in his environment to ensure predictability and avoid situations that are threatening to him. Individuals with fragile X can be operating at either end of this continuum, anywhere along the continuum, and in some instances at both ends of the continuum.

THE PROPRIOCEPTIVE SYSTEM

The proprioceptors are located in muscles, tendons, and joints, and are processed in the brain at the brain stem level. It is our proprioceptors that tell us when our body parts are moving and how far. This sense is sometimes referred to as kinesthesia. It is through proprioceptive awareness that we develop body scheme and body awareness. The ability to bend down and touch your toe without

looking is possible because of proprioception. When the proprioceptive system is not receiving or integrating information, it is difficult
to know where your body is or how to move it without the use of
vision. Children who have poor proprioceptive function are often
clumsy and have poor awareness of their bodies in relation to space.
They are often slow with tasks because, rather than having an automatic response, they need to use their vision and cognition to position the body and guide movement. In addition to this critical
function allowing us to feel and gauge movement, the proprioceptive system, along with the vestibular system, has an influence on
the entire nervous system. Inputs, provided by movement or by the
proprioceptive stimulation, have a calming and organizing influence
on the nervous system. In an attempt to reach this homeostasis, or
organized, productive state, individuals with sensory integrative
dysfunction (including many children with fragile X) seek out this
proprioceptive and vestibular input. Some common vestibular- and
proprioceptive-seeking behaviors are hand flapping, rubbing hands
together, biting hands, jumping up and down, rocking back and
forth, and others. The therapist must observe children and their behaviors and try to analyze the input and rationale. In general, slow
and rhythmic movements and behaviors are calming (inhibitory),
and fast-paced irregular movements are stimulating (facilatory). In
children with fragile X many of the unusual and often annoying
behaviors seen are not random and purposeless, but rather the
individual's attempt to provide himself with sensory organization.

VISUAL SYSTEM

Deficits in the ocular-motor system have not been as well documented in individuals with fragile X as deficits in other sensory
areas. Maino, Schlage, Maino, and Caden (1990) have described
visual problems in fragile X. It is reported that strabismus and
refractive errors occur more commonly in children with fragile X
than in the general population. A significant vision problem,
stabismus is reported to occur in up to 50% or more of the fragile
X population. Strabismus is when one of the eyes looks where it
should and the other eye is turned in (esotropia), out (exotropia), or
up or down (hyper- or hypotropia). The treatment of this condition
may include one or any combination of the following: prescribing of
eye glasses, patching, surgery, and vision therapy. Children and
adults with fragile X show a moderate to high incidence of refractive
error. These refractive errors include myopia (nearsightedness),
hyperopia (farsightedness), and astigmatism (blurred vision). If these

refractive errors are not corrected at an early age, amblyopia (lazy eye) may result in loss of vision in that eye. Refractive correction is most frequently achieved with eye glass prescription.

Other ocular-motor irregularities that may occur in fragile X are nystagmus (an involuntary, rhythmic back and forth movement of the eye ball), poor saccades (the ability to look from object to object), and poor pursuits (the ability to track a moving object). Impaired eye contact and gaze aversion, the most obvious fragile X behavior characteristics that seem to be related to the visual system, are most probably not a function of vision but rather manifestations of sensory defensiveness. Looking directly at someone or having someone look directly at an individual with fragile X may be perceived as threatening, so he protects himself by avoidance, much as happens with tactile hypersensitivity. Covering the eyes, another behavior often seen when visual input becomes overstimulating or overwhelming, is, again, a defense mechanism to limit overstimulation or fear of overstimulation.

AUDITORY SYSTEM

The auditory receptors are located in the ear and the input is processed in the auditory cortex of the brain. The auditory system has links to the vestibular system. Vestibular input is thought to enhance auditory processing, and in the child with fragile X, more appropriate verbalizations often accompany vestibular stimulation. (For more information on this connection, refer to Chapter 8.) Children with fragile X often engage in such stereotypic behaviors as covering their ears or becoming agitated and disorganized in the presence of intense or confusing auditory stimulation. These reactions indicate that many persons with fragile X are hypersensitive to input from their auditory channel. This disorganized sensory processing is also accompanied by significant problems in the area of auditory processing (discussed in Chapter 5). Frequent otitis media, or ear infection, may be the result of the connective tissue disorder and hypotonia that are common characteristics of fragile X.

OLFACTORY AND GUSTATORY SYSTEMS

The olfactory system is our sense of smell. Receptors are located within our nose and are processed at the cortical level of the brain. This system has close ties with our sense of taste as well as our emotions. Olfactory ties to the limbic system and to memory may cause primitive or nondiscriminating behaviors. One of the frequently observed behaviors in children with fragile X is the act of smelling of nonfood items. This response involving olfactory input is just one more example of a disorganized sensory processing system. Some individuals with fragile X have a very keen sense of smell, and, again, this may be considered a hyperresponse to a basic sensory input. This response becomes maladaptive when an individual cannot filter out the smell so he can pay attention to more pertinent input.

The gustatory system is our sense of taste. The receptors for this system are located in our mouths, primarily on the tongue. We have different receptors for such different tastes as sweet and sour. In the young child with fragile X, the need to "mouth" or taste objects seems to persist much longer than in nonfragile X children. This may be caused by delays in development, but could also be another indicator of need for additional input in an attempt to organize and control the sensory input. Oral input can also be used as a centering, calming, and organizing strategy, much as we experience when we chew gum or vigorously munch on a piece of hard candy, or as a baby uses a pacifier.

FEMALES WITH FRAGILE X

As is true with all other aspects of fragile X, the sensory motor characteristics of females are not as noticeable as in males. One reason for this may be that less than one-third of females affected have some degree of mental retardation. Many of the characteristics seen in boys with fragile X are also characteristics commonly seen in individuals with mental retardation. Problems most frequently cited in females are hyperactivity, attention deficit, and some stereotypic behaviors. Females show deficits in areas that suggest impairment of the nondominant hemisphere of the brain. Some of these deficits are in visual-spatial relationships, math ability, right/left orientation, and the area of constructional praxis. These are all characteristics that are also present in males with fragile X, but in males the effects of these deficits are usually compounded by cognitive impairment. The primary affected area in females is psychosocial.

THE EFFECTS OF MATURATION

There is no evidence that the sensory motor deficits of the child with fragile X actually lessen or go away as the child reaches adolescence or adulthood, but with treatment and intervention the behavior responses can be modified and changed. As the fragile X individual learns ways to gain control over his external environment and how this modifies his internal (sensory) self, the behaviors and responses do change. The individual can use socially acceptable ways to calm himself and remain in control. Some maturation of the sensory system may occur, but most changes occur externally as the child and his family use learned responses for inhibition and benefit from social development.

SUMMARY

This chapter has provided a review of the motor and sensory systems in the individual with fragile X syndrome. Within each system, the behavioral characteristics and the rationale for the most commonly observed behaviors are described. Some of the behaviors seen are a direct manifestation of a system that is not operating correctly, such as low muscle tone and poor postural mechanisms and auditory processing. Other behaviors seen are thought to be the individual's attempt to provide himself with the input he needs (for example, hand flapping at the time of sensory overload in an attempt to use proprioceptive input for inhibition or calming). The goal of sensory integration therapy is to enhance the efficiency of sensory processing. When and if this happens for a fragile X child, a more integrated system can lead to better organization and fewer defensive responses to daily experiences. Because this maturation or change in sensory processing can occur slowly or may not happen for many individuals with fragile X, it is paramount to be able to analyze the behaviors and recognize what sensory channels are involved. This helps the child recognize his need for external control and find a more socially acceptable way of providing himself with the needed sensory input for an appropriate adaptive response. Table 4-1 (see p. 70) provides a summary of the behavioral characteristics of fragile X individuals that are linked to deficits in their motor and sensory systems.

REFERENCES

Ayres, A.J. (1973). *Sensory integration and learning disorders.* Los Angeles: Western Psychological Services.

Clark, F.A., Mailloux, Z., & Parham, D. (1989). Sensory integration and children with learning disabilities. In P.N. Pratt & A.S. Allen (Eds.), *Occupational therapy for children* (pp. 359-405). St. Louis: C.V. Mosby.

Davids, J.R., Hagerman, R.J., & Eilkert, R.E. (1990), Orthopaedic aspects of fragile X syndrome. *Journal of Bone and Joint Surgery, 72A*(6), 889-896.

Fisher, A.C. (1991). Vestibular-proprioceptive processing and bilateral integration and sequencing deficits. In A.G. Fisher, E.A. Murray, & A.C. Bundy, *Sensory integration: Theory and practice* (pp. 71-107). Philadelphia: F.A. Davis.

Fisher, A.G., Murray, E.A., & Bundy, A.C. (1991). *Sensory integration: Theory and practice*. Philadelphia: F.A. Davis.

Levitas, A., Braden, M., Van Norman, K., Hagerman, R., & McBogg, P. (1983). Treatment and intervention. In R.J. Hagerman & P.M McBogg (Eds.), *The fragile X syndrome: Diagnosis, biochemistry, and intervention* (pp. 201-226). Dillon, CO: Spectra Publishing.

Maino, D.M., Schlarge, D., Maino, J., & Caden, B. (1990). Ocular anomalies in fragile X syndrome. *Journal of the American Optometric Association, 61,* 316-323.

Royeen, C.B. (1985). Domain specifications of the construct of tactile defensiveness. *American Journal of Occupational Therapy, 39,* 596-599.

Wilbarger, P., & Royeen, C.B. (1987, May). Tactile defensiveness: Theory, applications and treatment. Annual Interdisciplinary Doctoral Conference, Sargent College, Boston University.

ADDITIONAL READINGS

Ayres, A.J. (1979). *Sensory integration and the child.* Los Angeles: Western Psychological Services.

Braden, M.L. (1990, Fall). Maximizing the potential in fragile X adolescents and adults. *Fragile X Southeast Network Newsletter,* 1-2.

Burns, E., & Hickman, L. (1989). Integrated therapy in a summer camping experience for children with fragile X syndrome. *Sensory Integration, 17,* 1-3.

Hagerman, R.J., & Smith, A.C. (1983). The heterozygous female. In R.J. Hagerman & P.M. McBogg (Eds.), *The fragile X syndrome: Diagnosis, biochemistry, and intervention* (pp. 83-94). Dillon, CO: Spectra Publishing.

Hagerman, R.J., & Silverman, A.C. (1991). *Fragile X syndrome: Diagnosis, treatment, and research.* Baltimore, Johns Hopkins University Press.

Hickman, L. (1988). Sensory integration and fragile X. *Fragile X Association of Michigan Newsletter,* 6.

Hickman, L. (1989). Fragile X syndrome and sensory integrative therapy. *Sensory Integration International News, 17,* 14-15.

Miejejeski, C., Jenkins, E.C., Hill, A.L., Wisniewski, K., & Brown, W.T. (1985). A profile of cognitive deficit in females from fragile X families. *Neuropsychologia, 65,* 110-117.

Reiss, A.L., & Freund, L. (1990). Fragile X syndrome. *Biology and Psychiatry, 27,* 223-240.

Van Housen-Selley, K. (1987, Autumn). Insights into motor skills in fragile X syndrome. *Fragile X Foundation Newsletter,* 2-3.

TABLE 4-1. Behavioral Manifestations of Motor and Sensory Deficits

	MOTOR AND SENSORY SYSTEMS					
MOTOR	**VESTIBULAR**	**PROPRIOCEPTIVE**	**TACTILE**	**VISUAL**	**OLFACTORY**	**GUSTATORY**
scoliosis	low tone*	hand flapping	tactile defensiveness	poor eye contact	inappropriate sniffing and smelling	excessive mouthing
flat feet	inadequate postural responses*	jumping*	excessive need to touch materials	strabismus		drooling**
poor equilibrium reactions*	decreased auditory* processing	rocking*	preference for certain types of clothing	refractive errors	keen sense of smell	strong food preferences
hypotonia* poor balance*	ocular motor difficulties*	pacing*		astigmatism		
connective tissue dissorder	rocking*	hand biting	emotional outbursts*	poor ocular motor control		
		rubbing hands together				
toe walking*	jumping*	poor body awareness*	hyperactivity*	covering eyes		
oral motor deficits*	pacing*	toe walking*	poor body awareness*			
residual primitive reflexes	inflexibility		social withdrawal*			
hyperextensibility of joints	gravitational insecurity		toe walking*			
delayed development of gross motor skills	social withdrawal		fine motor delays*			
delayed development of fine motor skills*	poor balance*					
	inefficient equilibrium reactions					
delayed speech and oral skills*	clumsy					
	poor body awareness*					

** Also related to low muscle tone in the oral area.

* You will note that some characteristics are listed under more than one sensory or motor system. This is because often one system has influence on one or more other systems, and behavior cannot be neatly listed in only one area.

Note: Not all children with fragile X syndrome have all of these characteristics and the degree that any characteristic is present varies greatly from individual to individual.

BEHAVIORAL CHARACTERISTICS

5

SPEECH AND LANGUAGE CHARACTERISTICS IN FRAGILE X SYNDROME

Since the discovery of the fragile X syndrome, doctors, researchers, and clinicians have noticed a distinctive and unique pattern of speech and language characteristics associated with the disorder. Early references in the literature mention "jocular," "litany," and cluttered speech, as well as fast rate and poor intelligibility. Recent articles have begun to describe fragile X speech and language patterns and to compare them to other communicatively impaired populations, such as individuals with Down syndrome, autism, and other forms of X-linked mental retardation. In this chapter, the characteristics commonly observed in the speech and language of males with fragile X are discussed. Not all fragile X boys display all of these features, and the relative severity of the characteristics varies from individual to individual. As with any handicapped child, individual strengths and weaknesses are more important than diagnosis in determining treatment objectives. However, knowledge of the common profile of fragile X and the possible causative factors of some of the speech and language deficits is valuable to the clinician. Most significantly, the different speech and language characteristics are interrelated. This chapter and the last (sensory motor characteristics) provide a foundation upon which therapeutic programs may be built.

ORAL SENSORY-MOTOR SKILLS

Boys with fragile X syndrome usually show some dysfunction in oral sensory and motor skills. The sensory integration deficits in fragile X impact on the functioning of the oral area for eating and for speech. These deficits include abnormal sensory feedback in the mouth, low muscle tone, tactile defensiveness, and dyspraxia (problems with motor planning).

Sensory Deficits

The disturbed sensory processing system of the fragile X child may result in the mouthing of fingers and objects and in tactile defensiveness. Fragile X boys often put their fingers in their mouths, especially during unfamiliar or anxious situations. One study of the oral health of fragile X males (Shelhart, Casamassimo, Hagerman, & Belanger, 1986) found a significantly higher rate of crossbite and openbite in their subjects, which may be due to the habitual mouthing of fingers. A related behavior sometimes observed in this population is rubbing the face with saliva. These activities may provide calming sensory input to the child. Simko, Hornstein, Soukup, and Bagamary (1989) cite the mouthing of objects past a young age as a common behavior in fragile X males. Objects may be put in the mouth particularly often during times of stress or sensory overload. "Stress" for a child with fragile X may be more broadly defined than for individuals with normal sensory systems. Situations or events that would not normally be perceived as stressful may be overwhelming to children with fragile X. A change in routine, a direct question with a specific desired response, even eye contact may provoke anxiety, and the resulting behaviors may include mouthing of fingers or objects. Biting may be another oral response to stress. For example, during oral motor stimulation activities, a toothbrush may be bitten hard between the molars. Fragile X boys seem to particularly like this type of activity, perhaps because it provides calming proprioceptive input to the temporal-mandibular joint. The tendency to bite the hands, which is sometimes observed in fragile X (Hagerman, Amiri, & Cronister, 1991) may be related to the need for sensory input.

A second sensory-related behavior seen in fragile X boys is tactile defensiveness. At times the abnormal sensory system of the fragile X child appears hyposensitive—hence the need for the mouthing behaviors just discussed. Because the nervous system does not function normally, however, this hyposensitivity can rapidly become hypersensitivity, and the input that has been pleasurable can become aversive. Sensitivity can also vary depending on the type and source of the stimulation, as well as on the environment. For example, light touch vs. deep touch, and touch by a familiar vs. unfamiliar person are factors which influence tolerance of tactile input. The amount of other sensory stimulation occurring in the environment at a given time is also a factor in the ability of the fragile X individual to accept tactile input. Sensory input is discussed in detail in Chapters 4 and 6. Boys with fragile X frequently display tactile defensiveness throughout their bodies, and often it is especially apparent in and around the mouth. Braden (1989) includes "difficulty tolerating food textures" and "often pushes food or drink away" as items on her parent questionnaire. Hagerman et al. (1991) not only include tactile defensiveness as an item on the Fragile X Checklist, but also found it to be one of four traits statistically significant in distinguishing fragile X-positive and -negative patients. Fragile X children may be unwilling to eat foods with certain textures, such as crunchy, firm, or mushy. They may refuse to eat foods which have more than one texture, such as yogurt with granola, or raw vegetables with dip. They may also refuse to eat with utensils, because the fork or spoon in the mouth adds an additional texture which they cannot tolerate. In one case, a 7-year-old boy with fragile X required months of daily oral stimulation to build tolerance for more than one texture (a food plus a utensil) in his mouth. Even after this goal had been reached, however, he still reverted to finger feeding if the food presented had multiple textures. Tactile defensiveness in the oral area can affect not only eating but other routine activities such as tooth brushing, dental visits, and face washing. A study of oral structure, disease, and malocclusion (Shelhart et al., 1986) noted excessive gagging in their fragile X subjects, suggesting a high degree of oral tactile defensiveness. Hyposensitivity can result in continuous stuffing of food into the mouth before a previous bite is swallowed. Fragile X children appear to lack adequate sensory feedback, so that a full mouth is not always perceived. Fragile X children also tend to break up and play with their food while eating, probably also a sensory-related behavior. The chapter on speech and language intervention addresses techniques for normalizing sensitivity in the oral area.

Motor Deficits

Motor problems in fragile X boys include low muscle tone and motor planning problems, or dyspraxia. Low muscle tone in the oral area can result in reduced efficiency in handling food or liquids. Braden's (1989) parent questionnaire includes a query on difficulty drinking from a bottle as an early characteristic of children with fragile X. Lip closure may be inefficient, resulting in chewing with the lips open, poor lip seal on the rim of the cup, and generally "messy" eating. The combination of tactile defensiveness and low tone can lead to mealtime behaviors which look inappropriate and careless, although the cause is often physiological rather than behavioral. Low muscle tone in the tongue, lips, and cheeks may also affect intelligibility by causing less firm and precise articulatory contacts. Drooling may also be present in fragile X, as a result of both poor lip closure and inadequate sensory awareness of saliva in the mouth. Otitis media, a frequent problem with fragile X children addressed in this chapter's section on auditory problems, may be a result of low tone, which produces a floppier eustachian tube with less efficient drainage (Hagerman, Altshul-Stark, & McBogg, 1987).

A second motor deficit seen in fragile X is dyspraxia. Praxis refers to the planning of voluntary movement. Normal speech production requires rapid, smooth, sequential movements of the articulators, combined with appropriately timed respiration and phonation. Individuals with fragile X syndrome have difficulty with these skills (Hanson, Jackson, & Hagerman, 1986; Madison, George, & Moeschler, 1986; Paul, Cohen, Breg, Watson, & Herman, 1984; Scharfenaker, 1990; & Vilkman, Niemi, & Ikonen, 1988). Smooth praxis is interrupted, and children with fragile X show many of the characteristics of verbal dyspraxia. These characteristics include (Paul et al., 1984, p. 331):

1. Disfluencies consisting of prolongations and repetitions of sounds and syllables;
2. Adequate production of sounds and words in isolation, with connected speech less intelligible than would be predicted based on articulation testing;
3. Incorrect sequencing in tasks involving imitation of nonreduplicative syllables (puh-tuh-kuh);
4. Greater difficulty in the production of polysyllabic words than in one- or two-syllable words;
5. Greater deficits in expressive language than in receptive language.

Paul (1984, p. 331) states, "these characteristics may reflect an underlying impairment in the capacity for formulating and executing speech that is expressed across all levels of linguistic encoding." The specific speech and language problems included in this list of verbal dyspraxia characteristics are significant in the profile of fragile X males and are discussed in detail in subsequent sections and chapters of this book.

INTELLIGIBILITY

The intelligibility of fragile X males is affected by many factors, which are sometimes difficult to sort out. Most listeners find fragile X speech difficult to understand. Four major areas influencing intelligibility are articulation, prosody, fluency, and voice. Each is discussed separately, although the elements are very much related in their contribution to poor intelligibility. As with most features of fragile X syndrome, organizational divisions are artificial; the disorder is holistic, and diagnosis and treatment should always be approached from this perspective. For example, expressive language issues, discussed later in this chapter, affect the intelligibility of the fragile X speaker, but are not included in this section, which deals with more "speech-related" intelligibility factors.

Articulation

Fragile X boys often have a history of articulation problems. Usually these consist of substitutions of consonant sounds that tend to follow normal developmental error patterns. The high incidence of otitis media in childhood may be an influential factor in delayed speech sound acquisition. In several studies, the phonological skills of fragile X boys have been examined. The most common errors appear to be substitutions for /r/, /l/, /s/, /v/, and the voiced and unvoiced *th* (Paul et al., 1984; Prouty et al., 1988). Vilkman et al. (1988) found /r/ and /s/ to be the most difficult sounds for both fragile X and normal children. Vowel errors in fragile X speech were found by Vilkman to consist of omissions and substitutions. In 88% of the vowel errors, vowel height was off by one feature only. The authors of this study conclude that this proximity of error to target supports the influence of dyspraxia on the articulation of fragile X boys. Madison et al. (1986) observed that fragile X subjects who spoke in the longest sentences had the poorest intelligibility. This observation may be related to dyspraxia: longer sentences demand more complex motor sequences, which are prone to error in fragile X. In general, the specific phonological errors found in fragile X were similar to those found in normal young children. Palmer, Gordon,

Coston, and Stevenson (1988) found that the number of errors in articulation testing with fragile X children was most likely to relate to the youngsters' degree of mental retardation and amount of past speech therapy. They found no relationship between age and number of errors. We can conclude that the articulation errors of fragile X boys do not generally differ qualitatively from typical young children, and that quantitatively their errors reflect mental age and treatment.

Dyspraxia

The articulatory problems of fragile X speakers appear to be more related to dyspraxia, or underlying motor planning abilities, than to specific phoneme errors or process errors. Vilkman et al. (1988, pp. 218-219) state that "their phonological impairment does not seem attributable to peripheral articulation factors (dysarthria) but to a deeper part of language (motor encoding) . . . fragile X speakers are hypothesized to have a dyspractic speech motor problem which is partly related to developmental dyspraxia." The connected speech of fragile X individuals is usually much more difficult to understand than individual phoneme errors would predict. The characteristics of dyspraxia already discussed in this chapter provide an explanation for this observation.

Prosody

The prosodic features of language include rate, intonation and stress patterns, juncture, and rhythm. Prosody, as discussed by Hargrove, Roetzel, and Hoodin (1989) is important in intelligibility of speech because of its pragmatic and grammatic functions. Pragmatically, prosodic features influence how listeners interpret speech by focusing their attention, differentiating new from given information, and separating speech acts. Prosody also serves a grammatic function: for example, pauses signal important juncture boundaries, and falling intonation marks the ends of clauses and sentences. Prosody, therefore can be thought of as a factor that organizes communication for the listener's comprehension. The underlying dyspraxia of fragile X speakers influences their use of prosodic features, as well as sound production accuracy—further contributing to reduced intelligibility. Fragile X speech is characterized by rapid and uneven rate (sometimes described as staccato, explosive, or pressurized) and disturbed intonation, stress, and juncture (space between words). In the speech of fragile X boys, syllables are sometimes incorrectly stressed, the rhythm and intonation patterns of sentences are often inappropriate to the sentence content, and the spacing between words becomes lost in rapid-fire production. The inability to smoothly coordinate the motor sequences necessary for normal speech may be an important factor in the disturbed prosody of fragile X speakers. Prosodic features, especially rate, appear to be strongly influenced by the state of the individuals' sensory system at a given time. If the fragile X child is calm and relaxed, his rate of speech tends to be more normal. Techniques for using sensory integration principles as a strategy for improving speech intelligibility are discussed in the chapter on speech and language intervention, as is the use of imitation as a speech improvement strategy.

Fluency

Males with fragile X syndrome often have marked dysfluencies in their speech, most often described as cluttering, rather than stuttering, although some cases of stuttering have been reported (Palmer et al., 1988; Paul et al., 1984; Rosenberger, Wilson-Ciambrone, & Milunsky, 1982). Cluttering includes a fast and fluctuating rate and repetitions of sounds, words, and phrases (Hanson et al., 1986). Sound repetitions tend to occur randomly throughout the speech of fragile X males. Stutterers usually repeat initial sounds, syllables, or words, sometimes displaying silent blocks and facial grimaces, behaviors which do not seem to be part of the fragile X profile. Fragile X boys seem to be unaware of their cluttered speech (Hanson et al., 1986) and do not avoid situations, sounds, or words as stutterers may do. The dysfluencies in fragile X speech have a major impact on intelligibility and may be reduced by calming techniques (Chapters 6 and 7).

Voice

Fragile X children frequently have a distinctive voice quality. It has been described as hoarse or harsh (Palmer et al., 1988; Prouty et al., 1988), and seems to be breathy as well. The pitch has often been described as low (Palmer et al., 1988; Prouty et al. 1988), although when fundamental frequency was measured by Madison et al. (1986) it was found to be higher than average. Although voice differences are not a factor in intelligibility per se, they do contribute to the overall deviance of fragile X speech and may reduce clarity. The voice quality differences in fragile X may be physiologically related to low muscle tone in the laryngeal area. The volume, or loudness, of fragile X speech is often deviant as well. At least one author (Scharfenacker, 1990) reports increased loudness in fragile X speech. In our experience, boys with fragile X more often seem to have reduced loudness. In combination with their deficits in body orientation and eye contact discussed later, this soft, mumbling voice quality is a factor which negatively affects intelligibility. Also, uneven loudness is sometimes observed. A soft voice could be related to low muscle tone, causing reduced or inefficient breath support, or it could be related to dyspraxia, in that coordination of respiratory and laryngeal activity may be a problem. Or, it could be related to the anxiety produced by a social language situation. Again, it must be emphasized that the characteristics of fragile X speech and language are highly interrelated.

HEARING

Fragile X boys have been found to have a high incidence of otitis media prior to age 5. Hagerman et al. (1987) found that 63% of their 30 fragile X boys had six or more ear infections in the first 5 years of life. The hypothesized causes are a "floppier" eustachian tube, which may result from hypotonia and connective tissue dysplasia and/or the long, narrow face and high, arched palate characteristic of fragile X, which may cause subtle changes in the angle of the eustachian tube, in turn affecting fluid drainage from the middle ear. Whatever the cause, the frequent episodes of otitis media may exacerbate the cognitive, vestibular, speech and language, auditory perceptual, and behavioral problems seen in fragile X children.

In an investigation of auditory brain stem responses in fragile X, Arinami, Sato, Nakajima, and Kondo (1988) found that nearly half of their subjects had prolonged I-V Interpeak Latencies (IPLs). This type of IPL pattern indicates delayed conduction time in the neural pathways of the auditory system, supporting the theory of central rather than peripheral nervous system dysfunction. The authors of this study state that prolongation of IPLs can be related to early recurrent otitis media. For most fragile X subjects in this study, auditory brain stem response thresholds and peak latencies were normal, indicating normal detection of auditory signals. There is no evidence that school-age fragile X boys have higher than the normal incidence of conductive or sensorineural hearing loss, although cases of hearing impairment and deafness in fragile X have been observed.

PROCESSING OF AUDITORY INFORMATION

Auditory processing is the ability of the brain to attend to, discriminate, remember, and interpret auditory information. Fragile X boys are often described as having deficits in auditory processing (Fisher, 1991; Hanson et al., 1986; Scharfenaker, 1990). Poor attention, hyperactivity, and distractibility impact on the fragile X child's ability to process auditory information. The inability to screen out unwanted sensory input, as discussed in Chapter 4, contributes further to processing problems, as do over- and under-arousal of the sensory system and the susceptibility to sensory overload. This inability to process sensory input and the resulting behaviors are sometimes referred to as hyperreactivity. Fragile X boys sometimes cover their eyes while listening in an apparent attempt to improve processing by physically blocking competing stimuli.

Memory for auditory information is often relatively poor in fragile X when compared to general level of functioning (Howard-Peebles, Stoddard, & Mims, 1979; Madison et al., 1986; Scharfenaker, 1990). We have observed that while memory problems may exist for non-contextual, academic, and other externally imposed material, fragile X boys seem to have excellent retention abilities for humorous expressions and high-interest "intriguing" words, phrases, or topics. The perseverative and echolalic qualities of fragile X language, discussed later in this chapter, account in part for this observation. Unlike some children with these characteristics, fragile X boys usually produce their perseverative and echolalic speech in relatively appropriate contexts, frequently giving their expressive language a humorous cast. This ability to remember interesting information has implications for treatment which are discussed later.

The learning style of fragile X boys also influences their auditory processing abilities. As described in the chapter on cognitive skills, fragile X boys tend toward a simultaneous rather than sequential learning style. Information is more efficiently processed if it is presented as a whole rather than in sequential parts. In one case, an 8-year-old boy with fragile X syndrome was unable to attend to a story unless he was first told the ending. He apparently needed a sense of the whole story before he could attend to its parts. Semantic knowledge is related to simultaneous rather than sequential processing skills (Kirby & Robinson, 1987), and this may account in part for the relative strengths in vocabulary often shown by the fragile X child. Therapeutic techniques that capitalize on simultaneous learning are discussed in Chapter 7.

The anxiety connected to academic and social situations for fragile X boys may also interfere with their auditory processing abilities. In our experience with fragile X students, increases in repetitive language, gaze avoidance, and mouthing seem to be related to level of social demand, response requirement, situation familiarity, and amount of attention being focused on the child. As these stress factors increase, the ability to process auditory information appears to decrease. Treatment techniques can be designed to minimize anxiety. (See Chapters 6 and 7.)

RECEPTIVE AND EXPRESSIVE LANGUAGE

Authors who compare receptive and expressive language skills in fragile X speakers report results that may seem contradictory. Paul et al.(1987) found a trend toward poorer performance on expressive measures in a group of institutionalized adult fragile X males. Fisher (1991) and Wolf-Schein (1990) also say that expressive language is weaker than receptive, with receptive skills falling close to mental age. On the other hand, Madison et al. (1986) found expressive skills to be higher than receptive, probably reflecting use of automatic, imitated phrases and sentences. The disagreements among authors studying fragile X language can probably be explained on the basis of inexact definition of what aspects of language are being measured and how those aspects are defined. For example, "expressive language" may mean that grammar or length of utterance is measured without attention to whether or not content is meaningful. It seems important that future researchers and authors define exactly what parameters are being examined (Sudhalter, Scarborough, & Cohen, 1991).

Vocabulary

Many people who have studied or worked with fragile X children have remarked on their relatively high vocabulary knowledge and use. (Hanson et al., 1986; Scharfenaker, 1990; Wolf-Schein, 1990). This may reflect strengths in simultaneous processing. No published data are available concerning what specific types of vocabulary are learned most readily by fragile X boys, but our hypothesis is that high-interest or humorous words are among the most easily acquired. Boys with fragile X often use specific labels that seem to stand out from a "background" level of language which is more disorganized, dysfluent, and unintelligible. Largo and Schinzel (1985) state that some fragile X boys appear to have a changing, but not necessarily increasing, vocabulary. This observation supports the theory that some of the vocabulary strength of fragile X boys results from their echolalic and perseverative tendencies. Word retrieval problems are also a frequent observation (Scharfenaker, 1990; Sudhalter, Cohen, Silverman, & Wolf-Schein, 1990). Word retrieval is discussed further under Perseveration.

Grammar

Grammar is defined as morphology (word endings, tenses, plural markers, etc.) and syntax (the order in which words are combined to form sentences). Development of grammatic skills has been measured in the fragile X population in an effort to determine the relative strength or weakness of grammar as a language skill and its impact on other areas, such as deviant verbal behaviors. Levitas, Braden, Van Norman, McBogg, & Hagerman (1983) state that fragile X boys usually develop expressive language, including sentences, before 7 years of age, and that the language includes some echolalia but not much pronoun reversal. Paul et al. (1984) found low Developmental Syntax Scores (Lee & Cantner, 1971) in their fragile X subjects due to deficits in verb marking, embedded sentences, use of conjunctions, and interrogative reversals. The lack of interrogative reversals and conjunctions was common to all three subjects. Perhaps the lack of conjunction use is related to the short, explosive bursts which often compose the speech of the fragile X boy. Scharfenaker (1990) states that the verbal imitative abilities of fragile X boys may lead to relatively well-developed syntax in some instances; however, this may reflect rote usage rather than true generative grammar skills. Because syntax is related to successive, or sequential, rather than simultaneous processing (Kirby & Robinson, 1987), the relative weakness of the fragile X boy in sequential processing may partially account for the apparent delay in syntax. Receptive grammar knowledge should be studied in more detail to determine its relationship to expression.

Sudhalter et al. (1991) studied the expressive language levels of fragile X males in relation to the proportion of deviant repetitive language used. They found that the relationship of complexity to length in these fragile X speakers resembled that found in normal children of a younger age, and that the fragile X speakers' deviant repetitive language was not related to their syntactic level. This finding supports the theory that both deviance and delay are factors in the language of fragile X boys.

Language Organization

The simultaneous learning style of fragile X boys combined with their perseveration, dysfluency, and tangential language content creates difficulties in sequencing skills and in language organization. It is usually very difficult for fragile X boys to relate an event in sequence, even with visual cues. Scharfenaker (1990) cites sequencing as a deficit area in fragile X, and Hanson et al. (1986) refer to false starts and self-interruptions, plus difficulty with formulation, integration, and sequencing of ideas. They also refer to "informational redundancy" as characteristic of fragile X.

Excessive Verbalization

Many fragile X children show an inability to inhibit verbalizations, resulting in nearly constant speech production. They frequently talk to themselves, perseverate, repeat, or self-interrupt. Several factors may explain this high level of speech output: impulsivity, hyperactivity, poor motor planning, anxiety, lack of ability to judge the pragmatic constraints of the situation and to "read" social cues from others, and "time-buying" in order not to lose the listener's attention. Inability to be appropriately quiet may lead to obvious problems in a classroom or group instruction situation and may also interfere with auditory processing.

Perseveration

Perseveration is a frequently observed characteristic of fragile X language. It consists of inappropriate fixations on and repetition of words, phrases, or topics. Fragile X boys often perseverate on stereotyped phrases or interjections, as described by Paul et al. (1984). Their subjects each used a repetitive interjection: "rats," "pits," and "jeepers," respectively. Perseveration was found by Wolf-Schein et al. (1987) to be one of the language characteristics which differentiated fragile X subjects from IQ-matched subjects with Down syndrome. Other factors were the related characteristics of jargon, echolalia, inappropriate and tangential language, and talking to self. Difficulty with word retrieval may contribute to the tendency to perseverate: it may be an effort on the part of the fragile X individual to "hold the floor" while being unable to produce novel language.

Echolalia

Fragile X boys have been observed to display some echolalic tendencies, especially in the early stages of verbal language development (Largo & Schinzel, 1985; Levitas et al., 1983). Most authors mention echolalia in their descriptions of the characteristics of fragile X language deficits. An interesting observation by Levitas was that despite the echolalic behavior of fragile X boys, they showed little delayed echolalia and little pronoun reversal, which is often associated with echolalia in children with autism. Sudhalter et al. (1990)

found that when compared to boys with autism and Down syndrome, boys with fragile X produced more perseveration and less echolalia than did the boys with autism.

Conversation

Several authors have recently attempted to examine the conversation skills of fragile X boys. Sudhalter et al. (1990) found that fragile X males produced significantly more deviant repetitive language in conversation than did males with Down syndrome, but not as much as did males with autism. The amount of repetitive speech patterns produced by fragile X males may be related to the social conditions of the interaction: Cohen, Fisch, Sudhalter, Wolf-Schein, and Hanson (1988) report a relationship between occurrence of repetitive speech and whether the child initiated the conversation or was responding to a stranger. Ferrier (1987) also found that the conversational skills of fragile X boys differed significantly from those seen in Down syndrome and autism: the fragile X boys used the most eliciting utterances and the most partial self-repetitions. Turn-taking and topic maintenance are basic areas of conversational ability that are frequently problematic for fragile X boys. Hanson et al. (1986) found rapid and inappropriate topic changes, revision behaviors, and informational redundancy to be characteristic of this population, as well as tangential thinking and poor topic mainte-nance. Lord (1990) cites difficulty with joint attention as a char-acteristic of the social interactions of fragile X children and adoles-cents. She feels that the delayed language of fragile X boys affects their ability to determine the relevance of their own behavior and their ability to perceive others' intentions and topics of conversation. Certainly, the attention problems of fragile X boys impact on their conversational abilities. Problems initiating and maintaining a conversation appropriately appear frequently in fragile X, although their conversation does not seem to be as deficient as in children with autism (Sudhalter et al., 1990). The tangential style of thinking impacts on the ability of the fragile X child to answer direct ques-tions, especially on a first try. Some examples collected at Ivymount School are:

QUESTION	RESPONSE
"What's a good color for a horse?"	"Eyes"
"What should we put it in?"	"It's hot"
"I thought that coffee was for me"	"It's good"
"Can I have a spoon?"	"Coffee"
"How many people do you need to play Tic Tac Toe?"	"Jeffrey"

Another fragile X boy always preceded his answers with "I don't know," although he would then give the correct answer. This may reflect perseveration on a stereotyped phrase, word-finding problems, anxiety, or a combination of factors. Intervention for answering questions is discussed in Chapter 7.

The nonverbal conventions associated with conversation (eye contact, body proximity/position, and gesture) are often deviant in fragile X boys. Poor eye contact is frequently observed. Cohen et al. (1988) studied the social gaze patterns of a variety of groups. They concluded that the fragile X boys actively avoided social gaze, and that the avoidance could not be attributed to age, degree of language impairment, differential treatment by adult conversational partner, or familiarity with the adult. The fragile X boys did discriminate between parent and stranger, however, as did normal and Down syndrome subjects. The boys with autism and pervasive developmental disorder without fragile X did not show a difference in their gaze avoidance between parent and stranger. These results suggest a higher degree of social awareness on the part of the fragile X boys. Fragile X boys tend to show more gaze avoidance as they get older. In contrast, as autistic males get older and gain more communication skills, their responsive eye contact tends to improve (Cohen, Vietze, Sudhalter, Jenkins, & Brown 1991). An avoidance of eye contact suggests deliberate and selective behavior and a degree of social awareness. Gaze avoidance may be an outgrowth of the easily overloaded sensory system of the fragile X child: they may use this behavior in order to physically screen out input. A common observation by teachers and therapists working with fragile X students is that the fragile X boys respond to adult eye gaze by looking away, but then frequently return eye gaze when the adult looks elsewhere. This pattern was upheld in at least one research study (Cohen et al., 1989) and has implications for the physical arrangement of treatment sessions and the behavior of the therapists (Chapter 7).

Body positioning and proximity is often unusual in fragile X boys, a characteristic related to gaze avoidance. Instead of just averting their eyes, fragile X children often turn their whole heads or upper bodies away from their conversational partner. A study by Wolff, Gardner, Paccia, and Lappen (1989) described a stereotyped greeting behavior observed in fragile X males. The behavior consisted of turning the head and body away from the other person, while shaking hands and mumbling an appropriate verbal greeting. In subjects above age 12, 78% consistently showed this pattern. Although it was not observed in other mentally retarded groups, it was consistent in fragile X regardless of degree of retardation and social history. The behavior was displayed with all partners, including mothers and other fragile X individuals. Teachers often observe that fragile X students turn their bodies away even as they correctly answer questions.

The use of referential gesture, such as face and head movements and pointing, is often deficient in fragile X. Wolf-Schein et al. (1987) found lack of gesture use, possibly related to dyspraxia, to be a discriminatory factor between fragile X and Down syndrome groups.

SUMMARY

The fragile X male presents a unique profile of speech and language deficits and abilities that do not depend on cognitive level, although language delay is a factor in some areas, particularly grammar. The characteristics of the oral sensory-motor, speech, and language skills of fragile X males are:

1. Problems with oral sensation: mouthing, reduced awareness, drooling, tactile defensiveness, stuffing food;
2. Problems with oral motor function: low muscle tone, dyspraxia;
3. Difficulties with intelligibility: articulation, dyspraxia, fast and uneven rate, poor juncture, disturbed rhythm, hoarse and breathy voice, cluttering;
4. History of otitis media, unusual ABR latencies;
5. Problems with auditory processing;
6. Relatively strong vocabulary;
7. Delayed syntactic development;
8. Poor sequencing and language organization;
9. Excessive verbalizations;
10. Perseveration;
11. Echolalia;
12. Poor conversation skills: topic maintenance, turn-taking, tangential style, eye contact, body position, and gesture.

Many of these deficits exist in other groups of children with speech and language handicaps, and fragile X children vary greatly in their speech and language abilities. There seems, however, to be a characteristic, recognizable pattern of features in the speech and language skills of the fragile X child. Children displaying some or all of these characteristics should be tested for fragile X syndrome.

SPEECH AND LANGUAGE CHARACTERISTICS OF FRAGILE X FEMALES

Little information is available on the speech and language characteristics of fragile X females. Scharfenaker (1990) states that fragile X females often do not exhibit speech or language deficits. In cases where problems have been observed, the most common characteristics include problems with abstract reasoning, auditory processing, tangential language, and poor topic maintenance. Madison et al. (1986) report a conversational style characterized by a run-on narrative style, and revisions in 6-20% of phrases. In fragile X women with lower than normal IQ, speech content was inconsistently appropriate, and all the women used automatic phrases. The female subjects in this study also showed a below-average ability to repeat syllables on a timed motor task. Sobesky (1988) refers to disjointed, illogical thinking in fragile X females that leads to difficulty in communicating with others, poor eye contact, inappropriate laughing, and nervous body movements. Wolff et al. (1988) found that heterozygous fragile X females of normal IQ did more poorly than controls on measures of expressive language and auditory memory, while receptive language, visual memory, and naming abilities were equal. More information is needed about the abilities and disabilities of females with fragile X, which hopefully will be provided as diagnostic procedures become more easily available and accurate.

REFERENCES

Arinami, T., Sato, M., Nakajima, S., & Kondo, I. (1988). Auditory brain-stem responses in the fragile X syndrome. *American Journal of Human Genetics, 43*, 46-51.

Braden, M. (1989, April). Parent Questionnaire—Fragile X. International Fragile X Conference, Denver CO, (handout).

Cohen, I.L., Fisch, G.S., Sudhalter, V., Wolf-Schein, E.G., & Hanson, D. (1988). Social gaze, social avoidance, and repetitive behavior in fragile X males: A controlled study. *American Journal on Mental Retardation, 92*, 436-446.

Cohen, I.L., Vietze, P.M., Sudhalter, V., Jenkins, E.C., & Brown, W.T. (1989). Parent-child dyadic gaze patterns in fragile X males and in non-fragile X males with autistic disorder. *Journal of Child Psychology and Psychiatry, 300*, 845-856.

Cohen, I.L., Vietze, P.C., Sudhalter, V., Jenkins, E.C., & Brown, W.T. (1991). Effects of age and communication level on eye contact in fragile X males and non-fragile X autistic males. *American Journal of Medical Genetics, 38*, 498-502.

Ferrier, L.J. (1987). A comparison study of the conversational skills of fragile X, autistic, and Down syndrome individuals. *Dissertation Abstracts International, A: The Humanities and Social Sciences, 48,* 914.

Fisher, M.A. (1991). What is fragile X syndrome? Fragile X Association of Michigan, 1786 Edinborough Drive, Rochester Hills, MI, 48064.

Hagerman, R.J., Altshul-Stark, D., & McBogg, P. (1987). Recurrent otitis media in fragile X syndrome. *American Journal of Diseases of Children, 141,* 184-187.

Hagerman, R.J., Amiri, K., & Cronister, A. (1991). Fragile X checklist. *American Journal of Medical Genetics, 38,* 283-287.

Hanson, D.M., Jackson, A.W., & Hagerman, R.J. (1986). Speech disturbances (cluttering) in mildly impaired males with the Martin-Bell fragile X syndrome. *American Journal of Medical Genetics, 23,* 195-206.

Hargrove, P., Roetzel, K., & Hoodin, R. (1989). Modifying the prosody of a language-impaired child. *Language, Speech, and Hearing Services in the Schools, 20,* 245-258.

Howard-Peebles, P.N., Stoddard, G.R., & Mims, M.G. (1979). Familial X-linked mental retardation, verbal disability, and marker X chromosomes. *American Journal of Human Genetics, 31,* 214-222.

Kirby, J.R., & Robinson, G.L.W. (1987). Simultaneous and successive processing in reading disabled children. *Journal of Learning Disabilities, 20,* 243-252.

Largo, R.H., & Schinzel, A. (1985). Developmental and behavioral disturbances in 13 boys with fragile X syndrome. *European Journal of Pediatrics, 143,* 269-275.

Lee, L.L., & Cantner, S.M. (1971). Developmental syntax scoring: A clinical procedure for estimating syntactic development in children's spontaneous speech. *Journal of Speech and Hearing Disorders, 36,* 315-340.

Levitas, A., Braden, M., Van Norman, K., McBogg, P., & Hagerman, R.J. (1983). Treatment and intervention. In R.J. Hagerman & P.M. McBogg (Eds.), *The fragile X syndrome: Diagnosis, biochemistry , and intervention* (pp. 201-226). Dillon, CO: Spectra Publishing, Inc.

Lord, C. (1990). A cognitive behavioral model for treatment of social communicative disorders in adolescents with autism. In R.T. McMahon and R.D. Peters (Eds.), *Behavior disorders of adolescence: Research, intervention and policy in clinical and school settings* (pp. 155-174). New York: Plenum Press.

Madison, L.S., George, C., & Moeschler, J.B. (1986). Cognitive functioning in the fragile X syndrome: A study of intellectual, memory, and communication skills. *Journal of Mental Deficiency Research, 30,* 129-148.

Palmer, K.K., Gordon, J.S., Coston, G.N., & Stevenson, R.E. (1988). Fragile X syndrome IV, speech and language characteristics. *Proceedings, Greenwood Genetic Center, 7,* 93-97.

Paul, R., Cohen, D.J., Breg, W.R., Watson, M., & Herman, S. (1984). Fragile X syndrome: Its relations to speech and language disorders. *Journal of Speech and Hearing Disorders, 49,* 328-332.

Prouty, L.A., Roger, R.C., Stevenson, R.E., Dean, J.H., Palmer, K.K., Simenson, R.J., Coston, G.N., & Schwartz, C.E. (1988). Fragile X syndrome: Growth, development, and intellectual function. *American Journal of Medical Genetics, 30,* 123-142.

Rosenberger, P.B., Wilson-Ciambrone, S., & Milunsky, A. (1982). Speech fluency disorder in the fragile X syndrome. *Neurology, 32,* A190. (Presented at the 34th Annual Meeting of the American Academy of Neurology, April, 1982.)

Scharfenaker, S.K. (1990). The fragile X syndrome. *American Speech-Language-Hearing Association, 32,* 45-47.

Shelhart, W.C., Casamassimo, P.S., Hagerman, R.J., & Belanger, G.K. (1986). Oral findings in fragile X syndrome. *American Journal of Medical Genetics, 23,* 179-187.

Simko, A., Hornstein, L., Soukup, S., & Bagamery, N. (1989). Fragile X syndrome: Recognition in young children. *Pediatrics, 84,* 547-552.

Sobesky, W.E. (1988, Spring). Psychological problems of fragile X females. *The National Fragile X Foundation Newsletter,* 1-2.

Sudhalter, V., Cohen, I.L., Silverman, W., & Wolf-Schein, E. (1990). Conversational analyses of males with fragile X, Down syndrome, and autism: Comparison of the emergence of deviant language. *American Journal on Mental Retardation, 94,* 431-441.

Sudhalter, V., Scarborough, H.S., & Cohen, I.L. (1991). Syntactic delay and pragmatic deviance in the language of fragile X males. *American Journal of Medical Genetics, 38,* 493-497.

Vilkman, E., Niemi, J., & Ikonen, V. (1988). Fragile X speech phonology in Finnish. *Brain and Language, 34,* 203-221.

Wolff, P.H., Gardner, J., Paccia, J., & Lappen, J. (1989). The greeting behavior of fragile X males. *American Journal on Mental Retardation, 93,* 406-411.

Wolf-Schein, E.G., Sudhalter, V., Cohen, I.L., Fisch, G.S., Hanson, D., Pfadt, A.G., Hagerman, R.J., Jenkins, E.C., & Brown, W.T. (1987). Speech and language and the fragile X syndrome: Initial findings. *American Speech-Language-Hearing Association, 29,* 35-38.

Wolf-Schein, E.G. (1990). Fragile X syndrome. *American Speech-Language-Hearing Association, 32,* 55-56.

ADDITIONAL READINGS— SPEECH AND LANGUAGE

Cronister, A., Schreiner, R., Wittenberger, M., Amiri, K., Harris, K., & Hagerman, R.J. (1991). Heterozygous fragile X female: Historical, physical, cognitive, and cytogenetic features. *American Journal of Medical Genetics, 38,* 269-274.

Daker, M.G., Chidiac, P., Fear, C.N., & Berry, A.C. (1981). Fragile X in a normal male: A cautionary tale. *Lancet, 1,* 780.

Grigsby, J.P., Kemper, M.B., Hagerman, R.J., & Myers, C.S. (1990). Neuropsychological dysfunction among affected heterozygous fragile X females. *American Journal of Medical Genetics, 35,* 28-35.

Hagerman, R.J., Kemper, M., & Hudson, M. (1985). Learning disabilities and attentional problems in boys with the fragile X syndrome. *American Journal of Diseases of Children, 139,* 674-678.

Haldy, M. (1987, December). A summer day camp experience for children with fragile X syndrome: A case study. *Sensory Integration Special Interest Section Newsletter,* 2-3.

Laing, S., Partington, M., Robinson, H., & Turner, G. (1991). Clinical screening score for the fragile X (Martin-Bell) syndrome. *American Journal of Medical Gnetics, 38,* 256- 259.

McLaughlin, J.F., & Kriegsmann, E. (1980). Developmental dyspraxia in a family with X-linked mental retardation (Renpenning syndrome). *Developmental Medicine and Child Neurology, 22,* 84-91.

Newell, K., Sanborn, B., & Hagerman, R.J. (1983). Speech and language dysfunction in the fragile X syndrome. In R.J. Hagerman & P.M. McBogg (Eds.), *The fragile X syndrome: Diagnosis, biochemistry, and intervention* (pp. 175-200). Dillon, CO, Spectra Publishing, Inc.

Paul, R., Dykens, E., Leckman, J.F., Watson, M., Breg, W.R., & Cohen, D.J. (1987). A comparison of language characteristics of mentally retarded adults with fragile X syndrome and those with nonspecific mental retardation and autism. *Journal of Autism and Developmental Disorders, 17,* 457-468.

Wolff, P.H., Gardner, J., Lappen, J., Paccia, J., & Meryash, D. (1988). Variable expression of the fragile X syndrome in heterozygous females of normal intelligence. *American Journal of Medical Genetics, 30,* 213-225.

PART III

HOW DO YOU APPROACH INTERVENTION?

6

OCCUPATIONAL THERAPY FOR CHILDREN WITH FRAGILE X SYNDROME

Occupational therapy (OT) is based on the belief that purposeful activity may be used to prevent and mediate dysfunction and to elicit maximum adaptation. (American Occupational Therapy Association [AOTA], 1979). Mary Ann Fisher (1990), a parent of a fragile X child, states that occupational therapy is crucial for fragile X individuals because of their sensory and motor deficits (Chapter 4). The occupational therapist can be helpful in assessing and improving motor and sensory function in the child with fragile X, which can lead to more appropriate behavior and, thus, to greater availability to learn (Haldy, 1987). The nature of fragile X children's deficits suggests that the sensory integration principles developed by Dr. Jean Ayres can be used in OT as a framework for sensory motor therapy. Sensory integration (SI) treatment is considered a controversial topic that needs more research. As stated in the Preface to this book, we will not address the controversy other than to acknowledge its existence. The recommendation for using SI in therapy for fragile X children in based on our experiences and the opinions of other clinicians who have worked with this population. Readers should decide for themselves which treatment procedures help individual clients. Please refer to the special reference list at the end of this chapter, which provides further readings on SI efficacy studies.

SENSORY INTEGRATION THEORY

The sensory integration theory of the relationship of brain function and behavior is based on consideration of three important postulates. The first is that learning is dependent on the ability of the child to take in sensory information from the environment and from his body movements, to process and integrate this sensory input within his central nervous system, and to use this sensory information to plan and organize behavior. The second postulate follows from the first. If the child has deficits in processing and integrating sensory input, conceptual and motor learning suffer from loss of the ability to plan and act on productive behavior. Finally, the third postulate guides intervention. It hypothesizes that conceptual and motor learning will be enhanced by providing repeated opportunities for expanded sensory intake. Meaningful activities promote planning and organizing of adaptive behavior by improving the ability of the child's central nervous system to process and integrate sensory input (Fisher & Murray, 1991). If we are guided by this hypothesis, then it is implied that we need to focus on providing various types and amounts of sensory input in different contexts in order to increase learning potential for the fragile X child.

The theoretical framework for sensory integration was developed during the 1950s and continues with ongoing research today. Ayres (in Fisher & Murray, 1991) suggests that adequate early motor and sensory development leads to a well-functioning, mature organism able to perceive, integrate, and react purposefully to his environment. It is important to delineate the boundaries of sensory integration theory and practice before we can discuss using it as our frame of reference for treatment. We need to acknowledge that this theory is not intended to completely define the neuromotor deficits associated with fragile X, but that the approach, nevertheless, can provide a framework for treatment.

To clarify terms, the differences among sensory integration, sensory motor approaches, and sensory stimulation will be briefly explained. Sensory integration treatment techniques involve the use of enhanced, controlled sensory stimulation in the context of a meaningful, self-directed activity in order to elicit an adaptive behavior. Sensory motor approaches emphasize the application of specific sensory input, through handling or direct stimulation, with the goal of eliciting a desired motor response. In contrast to sensory integration, sensory stimulation involves the application of direct sensory input with the purpose of eliciting a more generalized behavioral response, such as increased attention or arousal, calming or decreased heart rate, or minimized depression. Sensory stimulation is a component of both sensory motor and sensory integration treatment, but, in itself, it cannot be considered to be either (Fisher & Murray, 1991).

A sensory motor therapeutic approach for a fragile X child is aimed at improving the child's interactions with the environment, facilitating the integrative and inhibitory processes, and aiding in development. Adaptive behavior goals should be established for the fragile X child, because he is faced with permanent sensory integrative dysfunction caused by neurological impairments.

The Sensory Integration Model as a Base for Sensory Motor Treatment

In the hierarchial process of sensory integration, the first therapeutic step is sensory awareness, or registration. At this level, a person orients to and perceives sensory stimuli from any of the senses—touch or tactile input, body sense, motion and gravity (or vestibular) input, gustatory, olfactory, visual, and auditory awareness (See Chapter 4). Goals for therapy focus on sensory registration and responsiveness levels. Specific goals are discussed later in this chapter.

The second step in the process of sensory integration involves sorting, organizing, combining, and processing information from the seven senses. At this stage, the brain integrates tactile, vestibular, visual, and proprioceptive messages to develop an awareness of body scheme. The brain acts as a filter to prevent constant bombardment by too much stimulation and by unnecessary sensory input, in order for attention to be focused on the tasks at hand. Other processes occurring as a result of this combining and redefining include reflex maturation, bilateral integration, praxis, and gravitational and postural security (Chapter 4). Therapy at this level focuses on helping the child seek out and use a carefully controlled and organized combination of types of sensory input to facilitate improved sensory processing within his central nervous system.

Once the sensory information has been taken in and processed, the foundations are in place for the third phase—developing perceptual motor skills, such as body coordination, eye-hand coordination, ocular motor control, visual spatial perception, postural adjustments, and auditory language skills. The most important brain function during the organizing and processing of sensory information from different channels is to make adaptive responses. Adaptive responses are purposeful, goal-directed responses to sensory experiences and are proof that the person is productively using his brain. To facilitate an adaptive response during therapy, the OT must challenge the child to explore, react, and discover something new.

A problem at any of the initial phases of taking in and processing information will affect higher level learning and thinking skills. In addition, the potential for emotional-social maturity is related to successful organization and development of sensory integration. When the brain is efficiently organizing, processing, and integrating sensory information, body movements are highly adaptive, learning is easy, and good behavior is a natural outcome. The final result is that new acquired skills are integrated into the whole functioning level of the child, instead of being isolated splinter skills. The child becomes a more productive member of society, able to deal with and function in the world around him.

It is important for the therapist to remember that all of our systems operate at different levels of efficiency. This is also true for the person with fragile X. At times of stress he will be more easily overloaded and become more hyperresponsive to stimulation. Every person has different strengths and weaknesses within his own sensory integration system. The differences between an ordinary person and someone who has sensory integration deficit, which in the case of fragile X is caused by neurological differences, is the effectiveness of a person's ability to function in the world around him. The person with fragile X is often unable to maintain a balanced level of responsiveness to sensory input and is more affected by stress. Before therapy can begin, the child must be evaluated thoroughly for his level of sensory motor functioning. The therapist must always observe and reassess the child's tolerance of environmental stresses before and during each treatment session.

The Evaluation

Sensory integration is evaluated using standardized tests, clinical observations, and information from parents and other professionals. The Sensory Integration and Praxis Tests (SIPT), by Ayres (1989), must be given by someone who is certified in its administration (Mailloux, 1990). Information concerning sensory integration may also be obtained from other tests and checklists, by supplemental observation during the testing, and by analysis of the quality of performance. Clinical observations can be made using tasks designed to look at the quality of adaptive responses. Such test information may be obtained using Ayres Clinical Observations (1973), A Guide to

Testing Clinical Observations in Kindergartners (Dunn, 1981), DeGangi-Berk Test of Sensory Integration (Berk & DeGangi, 1983), and by reviewing current literature and research on specific clinical observation items (King-Thomas & Hacker, 1987). Observation items include postural reflexes, cocontraction, muscle tone, extraocular muscle control, integration of both sides of the body, choreoathetoid movements, and ability to tolerate, screen out, and process a variety of types of sensory input. Vestibular processing is assessed by examining postrotory nystagmus and prone extension, and by observing the child's interactions with suspended equipment. Wiss and Clark (1990) conclude that, when used by trained, experienced therapists in conjuction with other standardized assessments and clinical observations, the Post Rotary Nystagmus test (Ayres, 1975), is adequately reliable and valid to provide unique information related to central vestibular processes. The researchers state that the test is designed as a measure of the central nervous system's diffuse processing of vestibular input rather than as a pure measure of vestibular function. Further useful observations of how the child with fragile X responds to touch and movement can be made by observing the child's performance on self-directed and therapist-directed sensory motor treatment activities. The Touch Inventory Evaluation (TIE), by Royeen and Fortune (1990), is a 26-item screening scale for determining tactile defensiveness in elementary-school-aged children. Educational team members may compile input that will provide a sensory motor profile of the child's level of functioning in and adaptability to his environment from a sensory processing perspective. (See Figure 6-1.)

Therapeutic Environment

Treatment is provided in a specialized environment by a trained occupational therapist. A well-equipped OT room will include a variety of types of suspended equipment and a scooterboard ramp for vestibular stimulation; a variety of brushes, lotions, and other tactile stimulation media; and a large selection of challenging and interesting play and motor development equipment. (Figures 6-2 & 6-3.) The room should be arranged to be inviting to a child, without being overstimulating. It should be sectioned into different work/play areas to meet his various and changing needs. It is important that the sensory environment be considered when planning therapy for the child with fragile X. Various equipment should be arranged to allow the child to choose and self-direct his therapy, when appropriate, while providing a safe space for treatment.

Figure 6-1. The Ivymount Affiliated Program for Therapy and Tutoring.

Sensory Motor History

Child's Name _____

In order to understand your child's needs, it is helpful to include your views of some specific behaviors or problems your child now displays or perhaps did display in the past.

Try to indicate how often the following behaviors occur(ed) by circling the appropriate letter in the left hand column:

N = NEVER   O = OCCASIONALLY   F = FREQUENTLY   C = CONSISTENTLY

Touch Sensation

N O F C   1. Seems bothered by going barefooted.
N O F C   2. Seems bothered by fuzzy socks and/or shirts.
N O F C   3. Seems bothered by turtleneck shirts.
N O F C   4. Dislikes the "feel" of new clothes or certain textures.
N O F C   5. Dislikes having face washed.
N O F C   6. Dislikes having hair washed or combed.
N O F C   7. Dislikes having nails cut.
N O F C   8. Dislikes playing on a carpet.
N O F C   9. After someone touches the child, he/she scratches or rubs the spot.
N O F C   10. Seems bothered by walking barefoot in the grass or sand.
N O F C   11. Dislikes getting dirty.
N O F C   12. Dislikes fingerpainting, playing in sand, paste or mud.
N O F C   13. Seems bothered when standing in line with other children.

Auditory Sensation

N O F C   1. Overly sensitive to sounds
N O F C   2. Needs directions repeated
N O F C   3. Misses some sounds and/or parts of conversations
N O F C   4. Confuses some sounds
N O F C   5. Likes to make loud noises
N O F C   6. Has lots of ear infections

Olfactory Sensation

N O F C   1. Overly sensitive to certain smells
N O F C   2. Ignores noxious or strong odors
N O F C   3. Difficulty discriminating odors
N O F C   4. Smells food, objects for exploration

(continued)

Figure 6-1. *(continued)*

Gustatory Sensation

N O F C   1. Overly sensitive to certain textures of food
N O F C   2. Overly sensitive to certain temperatures of food
N O F C   3. Acts as though all foods taste the same
N O F C   4. Mouths objects

Visual Sensation & Perception

N O F C   1. Has difficulty keeping eyes on objects
N O F C   2. Uses head movements when visually tracking
N O F C   3. Appears overly sensitive to light
N O F C   4. Rubs eyes or complains of headaches
N O F C   5. Closes 1 eye and/or tips head when looking/reading
N O F C   6. Becomes distracted by visual input
N O F C   7. Has difficulty discriminating colors, shapes, sizes
N O F C   8. Has trouble with puzzles
N O F C   9. Confuse foreground and background in pictures
N O F C   10. Reverse letters and/or words

Movement Sensation

N O F C   1. Seems fearful going up/down stairs, riding a teeter-totter, going on a swing
N O F C   2. Gets sick in cars, elevators, rides or planes
N O F C   3. Dislikes trying new movement activities
N O F C   4. Prefers fast moving or spinning activities such as carnival rides, roller coasters, etc.
N O F C   5. Likes/liked being tossed in the air
N O F C   6. Does not catch self easily when falls

Muscle Strength

N O F C   1. Slouches when sitting or standing
N O F C   2. Grasps objects too tightly
N O F C   3. Tires easily
N O F C   4. Seems weaker or stronger than average
N O F C   5. Moves slower or faster than other children

Coordination

N O F C   1. Seems accident prone
N O F C   2. Seems clumsy
N O F C   3. Falls, trips, bumps into things
N O F C   4. Difficulty hopping, skipping, running
N O F C   5. Moves entire body instead of turning head

(continued)

Figure 6-1. *(continued)*

Fine Motor Coordination

N O F C   1. Switches hands during fine motor tasks
N O F C   2. Difficulty manipulating small objects or tools
N O F C   3. Unusual pencil grasp
N O F C   4. Makes strokes too heavy or too light
N O F C   5. Makes letters of inconsistent sizes
N O F C   6. Has trouble staying within the lines on the paper
N O F C   7. Has trouble discriminating between upper and lower case letters
N O F C   8. Organizes papers poorly
N O F C   9. Difficulty with zippers, snaps, buttons

Please circle all that applies to your child:

Distractable	Poor Handwriting
Overly Active	Loses place when reading
Short Attention Span	Poor right/left discrimination
Poor self-confidence	Poor understanding of time concepts
Cries easily	
Very shy	Wears glasses for _____
Aggressive (at times)	Wears hearing aids

An integrated program involves planned carryover from the treatment room into the classroom, consultation, team meetings, and regular inservicing for other professionals and parents to increase their understanding of how a sensory integration framework operates. The occupational therapist needs to have training in theory and methodology of delivering sensory motor treatment designed to enhance sensory integrative functioning. The position of the American Occupational Therapy Association (1986) is that an occupational therapist who chooses to apply the principles and concepts for the mediation of sensory integration dysfunction should receive advanced training. Advanced training provides the therapist with the knowledge base necessary to identify dysfunction and develop specific occupational therapy programs.

The role of the OT will differ slightly depending on the type of service delivery model and the role of other members of the child's treatment team. In an educational setting, the primary function of the therapist is to facilitate classroom performance and learning. This may mean that many calming techniques are needed for the child with fragile X to function optimally in the classroom. In any given

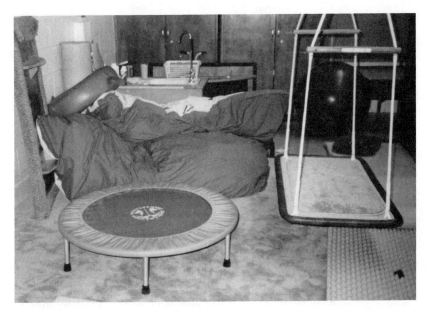

Figure 6-2. Occupational therapy equipment.

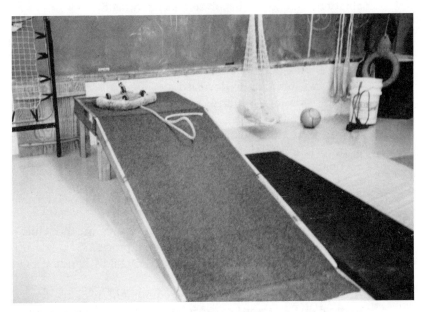

Figure 6-3. Ramp, scooterboard, and net swing for vestibular input.

situation, the primary focus may be the child's foundational skill development and daily living skills, or education of various members of the child's team on how to provide the sensory motor activities needed to influence behavior and adaptive responses. When formulating a treatment plan for the child with fragile X, one must look at the role other team and family members can play in influencing changes, in addition to evaluating the child's need for therapy. When scheduling the treatment, consideration should be given to other events that day or week, plus before and after the intervention, and how the child's overall schedule will affect change. When priorities must be set for the type and timing of services to provide, there are ten basic factors to guide the decision-making process (American Occupational Therapy Association, 1987, pp. 9.1-9.8):

1. How critical is it to the child's health and safety for the occupational therapist to be involved in providing services?
2. How much expertise and time of the occupational therapist will be needed to communicate adequately (verbally and in writing) with outside professionals?
3. How much will the occupational therapist have to contribute to environmental changes that improve the child's ability to function in his present environment?
4. How much do problems in sensory, perceptual, and motor processing interfere with the child's ability to function in his environment?
5. What is the potential for this child to improve functional skills and ultimately decrease or eliminate the need for special services of any kind, especially those of the occupational therapist?
6. Considering the child's chronological age, how might age-appropriate social demands affect the child's need for occupational therapy services and his ability to function independently?
7. Are other adults in the child's environment knowledgeable enough to carry out required activities?
8. What is the availability of other persons in the child's environment to assist in the educational process?
9. What is the level of interference of the child's handicapping condition?
10. Are appropriate space, time, and equipment available for the occupational therapist to carry out programs and services?

Providing occupational therapy services using sensory integrative principles to a complex child, such as a youngster with fragile

X, is an art form which requires training, experience, and skill (Scardina, 1981). The therapist's role in treatment is to control and organize the input a child receives and to develop a prescriptive environment to maximize the child's level of sensory integration. The OT must be a vigilant observer and use constant activity analysis to effect changes. She is responsible for finding ways to elicit adaptive responses that gradually extend the child's levels of functioning. The therapist may find it easier to use a holistic approach, because sequencing multi-step tasks is very difficult for the child with fragile X. It is important to teach functional skills the way you want the child to perform them the *first time;* do not use close approximations. The fragile X child often perseverates on the first response taught and also may tend to learn part of a multi-step response as the whole.

The therapist cannot organize the child's brain for him, or prevent or fix perseverations and sensory processing deficits; the child must make any changes possible for himself. Thus, the child's level of motivation and cooperation for the activity and for changing his level of functioning is of major importance. The art of therapy requires empathy and bonding with the child, the ability to construct an appropriate environment, and advanced knowledge of both neurophysiology and sensory integrative theory (Devereaux, 1984). The child is responsible for seeking out and making the adaptive responses himself for changes to happen. Therapy activities that are child self-directed will focus on areas of need. It is important for the therapist to remember that the activities are not the therapy. How the activities are applied to the needs of the child, based on the judgment of the therapist, composes the therapy. Activities must involve full body movement, including a complete range of types and intensities of sensory input, and also must enable the child's adaptive responses to be successful.

Goal Development

Once the child has been evaluated, and his strengths and weaknesses determined, it is time to develop the OT intervention plan which includes an Inidividual Education Plan and specific OT goals. The first step is to formulate long-term expectations. For the child with fragile X, goal areas to be covered include daily living skills, visual motor, and sensory motor goals as needed. The goals listed below are taken from the *Databased Individual School Curriculum* (DISC) manual developed at Ivymount School (Novakovich, 1989). This is part of a computerized IEP program. Goals are chosen as needed from the following menu:

1. Student will demonstrate improved daily living skills to care for self independently (Novakovich, 1989, p. 15).

The first area to be discussed is one that may be included in the child's educational or home program, or the OT may be responsible for working on the child's activities of daily living skills (ADL). This general area includes specific goals for eating and meal organization, toileting, clothing care, hygiene, managing work and leisure time, household management, community services, health, and career and prevocational skills.

2. Student will demonstrate improved visual motor, prehandwriting, and handwriting skills (Novakovich, 1989, p. 90).

This includes reading readiness skills such as visual attending, ocular motor control, and posture. Fine motor skills include developing and refining more mature grasp and release patterns, in-hand manipulation, establishing a dominant and helper hand, eye/hand coordination for manipulation tasks, and tool use including typewriter and computer skills. Handwriting goals include being able to reproduce forms, shapes, and designs, and reproducing legible letters and words in manuscript and cursive. Visual perceptual goals focus on discriminating objects, pictures and symbols, figure-ground and visual closure, directionality, visual memory and visual sequential memory, and spatial skills. Because of the educational nature of these goals, the therapist will need to coordinate with the child's teacher.

3. Student will demonstrate sensory motor and neuromotor foundations necessary for performing appropriate play, readiness, academic, and independent living skills (Novakovich, 1989, pp. 73-82).

Since this area is the bulk of the OT program, this goal is broken down into specific short-term objectives for purposes of this book as follows:

> Student will discriminate and organize sensory input necessary for focusing on and attending to classroom and therapy lessons. Student will maintain stable body positions as a base for movement and manipulation in order to complete classroom and therapy lessons.
>
> Student will improve components of normal movement patterns necessary for assuming and changing posture appropriate for classroom and therapy performance.
>
> Student will demonstrate improved oral motor control for eating and speech.
>
> Student will demonstrate awareness of body position and location in space while performing academic/therapy tasks involving stationary and dynamic positions.

Student will improve bilateral integration for efficiency and accuracy during movement and manipulative tasks in the classroom and therapy.

Student will perform isolated/segmented movements of hands, legs, head, and trunk for greater accuracy in classroom and therapy activities.

Student will make appropriate balance and postural adjustments to assume and change positions as needed during classroom and therapy activities.

Student will plan, sequence, and execute motions with ease, speed, and accuracy in order to follow teacher and therapist directions.

Student will increase physical strength and endurance in order to benefit from the therapy and classroom program.

Student will use sensory motor information in order to effectively plan and carry out functional living skills.

Student will use appropriate grasp, release, and in-hand manipulation patterns in manipulative, academic, and functional lessons.

These short-term objectives are also used by the physical therapist if the child is involved in an early intervention program, or if a physical therapist's services are specifically warranted. Under each short-term objective is a myriad of interim objectives listed in developmental order. In development of an IEP, strategies and criteria are chosen, duration and frequency are noted, and prioritized goals are selected. The criterion for measuring change may include performance on a specific test or test item or on a therapist checklist. If a therapist chooses to use a checklist, it should include performance in the child's natural environment as well as in the treatment room.

TREATMENT FACTORS

Phase One: Sensory Registration

Intervention should address the seven types of sensory input that can be explored during therapy to facilitate improved sensory registration and processing—touch, proprioception, movement, vision, audition, gustation, and olfaction. Each therapist must come up with her own creative adaptations that challenge the individual she is treating to seek out, participate in, and adapt to the various types and combinations of available sensory input in new and useful ways.

Tactile Input

Basic Goals.   A therapist provides tactile input to a child in order to facilitate that child's ability to feel motion, learn about his body, decrease tactile defensiveness, decrease fretfulness and aversion to touch, reduce hyperactivity, learn about the world at large, prepare the body to learn from other exercises, and facilitate movement (Jarek & Bell, 1978).

Goals for therapy include (Novakovich, 1989 p. 73):

- Indicate awareness of tactile input.
- Demonstrate increased tolerance of tactile input.
- Seek out appropriate stimulation.
- Decrease tactile self-stimulation.
- Localize tactile input.
- Identify a variety of familiar objects by touch.
- Discriminate various types of tactile stimulation.
- Demonstrate compensatory responses for inadequate tactile processing.

Another goal that is important for fragile X children is to utilize tactile information to facilitate functional activity.

Principles for Treatment.   The first stage of treatment involves gauging the degree of sensitivity, hypersensitivity, and responsivity levels. Does the child use the tactile information in a discriminating fashion to learn about his environment, or in a protective fashion? Therapy is designed to promote discriminatory touch. Because this kind of stimulation may not be tolerable for the fragile X youngster, the first focus of treatment must address increasing the child's tolerance for, and modulation of, touch. The various skin touch receptors sense vibration, touch-pressure, sharp input or pain, crude touch, temperature, light touch, and movement across the skin. The therapist must first prepare the child by providing vestibular stimulation, firm pressure, or proprioceptive input as needed for the child to accept and use touch input. The second part of therapy involves decreasing his arousal. The therapist must constantly evaluate how the child reacts to a given stimulation and control or avoid touch that is irritating. The third part of therapy involves increasing self-initiated tactile exploration. Motivation to explore touch input enhances the child's discriminatory system. Touch discrimination includes processing the touch for size, form, and texture information, and involves good in-hand manipulation skills to maneuver an object. Therapeutic activities for improving discrimination skills include identification and differentiation of textures and objects.

Tools and Therapeutic Techniques. Tools for providing tactile therapy may include brushes, feather dusters, cloth, creams and lotions, ace bandages, vibrators, therapy balls, pillows, a plastic pool filled with lightweight balls, raw rice, dried beans, or macaroni noodles. A tactile box should be assembled that includes a wide variety of different textures for the therapist and child to explore together (Figure 6-4). Games and songs should be developed to promote play and exploration that challenge, motivate, and promote creativity. Other activities that the teacher or therapist may use include art projects, cooking with different ingredients, and going barefoot on different textured surfaces, plus water and sand box play. Tactile input can be an inherent part of any activity by simply providing a textured surface on equipment the child will touch. An advantage to this is that the child is more likely to initiate the tactile stimulation himself (Figure 6-5).

Tactile input therapy should be provided early in the treatment session to diminish adversive responses to sensory input and allow greater contact with a sensory-defensive child. Early provision of

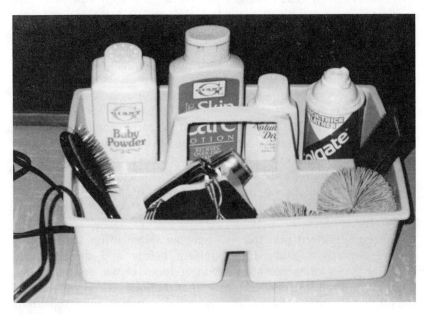

Figure 6-4. Tactile box.

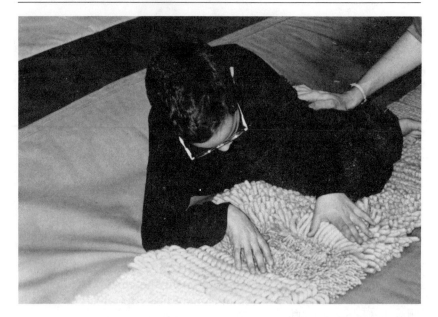

Figure 6-5.   Tactile stimulation using varied textures.

tactile input inhibits the fight or flight reactions of the parasympa-thetic nervous system (changes of involuntary body functions like sweating, increased heart rate, and changes in breathing patterns and skin color). Through tactile input therapy, the child's central nervous system achieves parasympathetic balance, and he is available for a greater duration and for greater amounts and types of sensory input. Combining touch input with bombardment of proprioceptive input appears to modulate the fragile X child's tactile responses and decreases defensiveness. Provide tactile stimulation to various areas of the body where many receptors lie, including hands, face, and forearms. Avoid stimulation against the grain of hair growth on the skin and avoid crossing the midline when brushing or rubbing unless you have determined the child is open to it. Tactile stimulation becomes contraindicated if a child's activity has increased beyond a desirable level; at that point it would only lead to further arousal.

Three important principles to remeber when using tactile input during therapy include: firm rubbing before and during more aversive types of tactile stimulation reduces tactile defensiveness; touching oneself is less threatening than being touched by another person; and anticipated touch is usually better tolerated than unexpected input. The therapist should keep in mind that tactile stimulation can have a cumulative affect on the child's nervous system, and watch for delayed and diffused reactions to the touch input.

There are various massage techniques that may be applied alone or in combination with lotions, oils, or creams. Massage techniques are effective in calming the child with fragile X by providing steady rhythmic movement over the child's body in a set pattern, usually distal to proximal. The therapist should be careful to use firm, slow, consistent movements. For example, stroking with fingertips of both hands along the spine from the nape of the neck to the top of the hips is done in continuous motion. Further training on the art of massage is suggested before the process is incorporated into treatment.

Other calming techniques employing tactile input include wrapping the child with ace wraps or blankets and allowing him to crawl in or under a large cloud (foam blocks sewn inside a casing made of sheets) for neutral warmth. The child may be given a vibrator or vibrating pillow to hold or squeeze, or even an electric toothbrush to play with. Lois Hickman (Scharfenaker, Hickman, & Braden, 1991) recommends using only natural fibers when choosing fabrics and objects which will come in contact with the child with fragile X. Ayres (1973) states that touch pressure is especially effective in modulating the child's response to tactile input. Grandin (1988) suggests using cloths of various textures ranging from soft velvet to coarse terry cloth, as well as standard paint brushes to apply touch-pressure input as the child is able to tolerate it. Playing in a pool of small balls is another effective way for the child to apply touch-pressure himself. When Krauss (1987) investigated the use of a hug machine for its deep touch pressure she found it had a positive effect. The touch pressure received through confinement had a calming affect by reducing the proprioceptive flow to the central nervous system and decreasing arousal through neurophysiological pathways and mechanisms.

The Wilbarger brushing program (Wilbarger & Royeen, 1987) is a new treatment program for sensory defensiveness which is a modification of Rood's technique (Ayres, 1973). Wilbarger's program uses surgical scrub brushes in conjunction with gentle joint compression to the upper and lower extremities and trunk in an intensive daily schedule. This type of brushing is effective as a preparatory activity for therapy, as well as a tool during therapy for calming and organizing the child's nervous system. It may also be used in combination with other intervention techniques. The intensive application schedule may be altered to fit the child's needs. Brushing is done by applying firm, quick strokes up and down the extremities followed by passive joint compression at all joints on that extremity. Ayres (1973) made the following statement which seems to apply to such a treatment regimen:

> Occasionally a therapist may be justified in applying stimuli in spite of discomfort for a few days in an effort to bring about a sufficient shift in balance between the protective and discriminative response systems to enable development of tolerance to some stimuli. If discomfort is still critical after a few weeks, the therapist is advised to reconsider the situation and remember that there is still much to be learned about the tactile system. (pp. 117)

Neurodevelopmental treatment (NDT) (Blanche & Burke, 1991a & b) and myofascial release (Lawton-Shirley & Wanzek, 1986) are tactile-based treatment techniques designed to facilitate improved function and motor output. The therapies employ sustained light pressure, sustained deep pressure, intermittent touch, slow and fast movement across the skin such as tapping and sweeping motions, and compression and traction to facilitate motion, posture, and muscle tone. It is important to remember that these are treatment techniques that employ the use of touch as a strategy, and should not be used if the child cannot tolerate tactile input, which is often the case for the child with fragile X. These techniques all require advanced training.

Compensatory Strategies.   Compensatory strategies for dealing with hypersensitivity to touch include providing a larger personal space in group activities, preparation before the activity, use of firm pressure as opposed to light touch during handling, and increased awareness and avoidance of noxious stimuli by the child. Preparatory activities include brushing, applying lotion, and other organizing (Tutterow, 1988) and calming strategies (Hickman, 1988; Van Hausen, 1987).

Proprioception

Basic goals.   A therapist provides proprioceptive input to the child in order to give the child information about where his body is in space, tell where one body part is in relation to another, develop the ability to automatically move through space, develop the ability to move one body part in coordination with another smoothly and efficiently, improve postural stability and gravitational security, decrease aversion to handling and moving, provide a calming influence on the child, and facilitate changes in muscle tone and movement.

Goals for therapy which focus on how the child handles proprioceptive input include (Novakovich, 1989, p. 73):

• Indicate awareness of proprioceptive input.
• Decrease excessive proprioceptive self-stimulatory input.
• Utilize proprioceptive input to facilitate functional activity.

Another goal for the fragile X child is to compensate appropriately for inadequate proprioceptive processing.

Principles for Treatment.   Proprioceptive input is received through the muscles, tendons, and joints and may be passive or active. Passive proprioceptive input techniques include passive range of motion (PROM), traction, and joint compression. The proprioceptive stimulation occurs when the child weight bears on an extremity or uses muscle contractions and cocontractions to either maintain or change his position. Joint traction and compression, especially to the small joints in the neck, wrist, and hand, are techniques that require advanced therapist training to avoid serious injury to the child. The activity may be part of a warm-up activity combined with tactile input, in which the therapist or child applies pressure to key body parts, such as the head or shoulders, to prepare the child for further therapeutic activities. The input may be given directly by the therapist, such as the joint traction and compression given during a massage or with myofascial release handling techniques; self-applied by the child by pressing or pulling on his own arms and legs; or may occur as a result of the child passively being moved across equipment such as therapy balls, wedges, or rolls, or by carrying heavy equipment or wearing weights or a weighted vest.

Active techniques include active range of motion (AROM) and the child's movement in his environment. Strong contraction of muscles and good cocontraction of body parts provides the child with proprioceptive input, which helps him interpret vestibular input. Examples of activities which provide increased proprioceptive input include jumping on a trampoline, bouncing on a hoppity-hop, pulling theraband (strips of rubber with graded degree of resistance), and using arms for propelling in a swing or on a scooter board.

Tools and Techniques.   Games and songs that include crawling, jumping, bouncing, hopping, and crashing present natural encouragements for the child to self-direct movement involving lots of proprioceptive input. Input is also stimulated through such functional activities as gardening, cooking, and art projects (like leather or woodworking) requiring heavy work such as pounding, pulling, pushing, and kneading.

Proprioceptive input is an important component in many calming and organizing activities done during treatment including rolling the child up in a foam mat or heavy blanket (hot dog roll), or making a "sandwich" by squeezing the child between two pillows or "clouds" to apply pressure to his muscles and joints (Figure 6-6). Another way to incorporate calming and organizing input into treatment is by having the child crawl inside a small barrel or box to work on fine motor or tactile activities. This may be used as a warm-up, but is always combined with other sensory input during therapy for the child with fragile X.

Compensatory Strategies.   Compensatory strategies for helping the child cope with his increased need for proprioceptive input include an exercise or self-range of motion (ROM) program so that the child may learn to apply pressure and weight to his joints and muscles himself. Such exercises include chair push-ups; squeezing or hugging; applying pressure downward on his own head, shoulders, arms, or knees; leaning on a table top or wall with extended

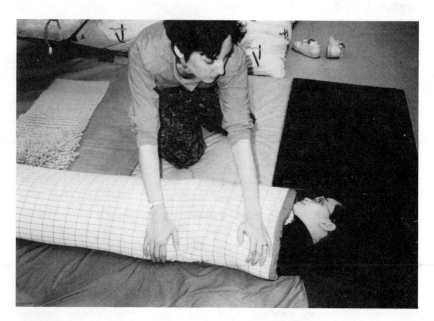

Figure 6-6.   Hot dog roll for proprioceptive input.

arms; and rocking on all fours. Careful determination of the appropriateness of such activities is needed, as the child may need to use the exercises outside of the treatment room. All movements provide the child with some proprioceptive input. However, the child with fragile X needs an increased amount of proprioceptive input due to his body scheme, motor planning, and sensory processing deficits in order to function in his environment and handle stress more appropriately.

Vestibular Input

Basic goals.   Vestibular input is provided through motion, vibration, and gravity and is received through receptors in the inner ear. The information is channeled to many different parts of the brain to influence development in all areas. Ayres (1973) said of the role of vestibular input in intervention, "Vestibular stimulation is one of the most powerful tools available for therapeutic use in the remediation of sensory integrative dysfunction" (p. 119.)

A therapist provides vestibular input for the child to develop automatic awareness of body in space, improve coordination of body movements, maintain balance, normalize muscle tone, decrease hyperactivity, increase eye control and visual skills, increase auditory alertness and language production, improve attending skills, and reduce stress.

Goals for therapy (Novakovich, 1989, p. 73) which focus directly on how the child handles vestibular input include:

- Indicate awareness of vestibular input.
- Demonstrate increased tolerance of vestibular input.
- Seek out appropriate vestibular stimulation.
- Demonstrate normalized response to vestibular input.
- Demonstrate the ability to assume and maintain the antigravity postures: prone-extension and supine flexion.
- Demonstrate improved postural security.
- Decrease vestibular self-stimulatory input.
- Demonstrate adequate response to vestibular input for functional activities.

Principles for Treatment.   Vestibular input can be described by how it is applied, plus the speed and direction of movement. Passive vestibular stimulation is applied by an external force, such as the therapist swinging or spinning a child. Active stimulation should be sought out and controlled by the child, thereby increasing the tactile and proprioceptive input incorporated into the activity. Both types of movement can be applied in a linear, orbital, or rotational direction, with the child's inner ear receptors positioned horizontally, vertically, or inverted. In addition to fast or slow movement, speed can be accelerating or decelerating. Different types of movements stimulate different receptors.

Tools and Techniques. Vestibular stimulation is applied every time and place that the child moves or is moved. However, to effectively provide vestibular input as a part of therapy, suspended equipment is required, so input may be applied in a variety of ways and directions to meet the many needs of the child with fragile X. Swings come in a variety of different shapes and sizes, including tire swings, platform swings, net swings, disc and bolster swings, helicopters, and rocket ships (Figures 6-7 & 6-8). Please note that the swings have many different names and applications. Some therapists are even able to design their own suspended equipment using commercial equipment in various combinations. Adaptations can be supported with a Bungee cord for more bounce, or other gross motor play equipment can be designed to suspend for more

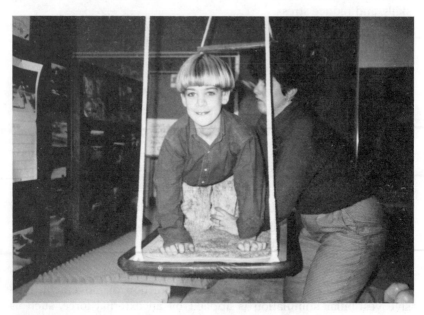

Figure 6-7. Platform swing for vestibular input.

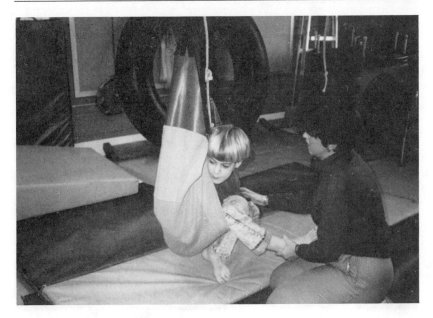

Figure 6-8.   Net swing for vestibular input.

movement. All equipment should be used with a safe, dependable provide the opportunity for changing speed and direction.

The child's reaction to vestibular stimulation is measured by ex-,amining his comments, behaviors, postrotary nystagmus, skin tone and color, autonomic nervous system reactions, and adaptive responses. The therapist should beware of the latent and cumulative effects of vestibular stimulation when planning for, providing, and observing vestibular input in combination with other types of sensory input. Caution is needed in applying vestibular input when working with a child who has heart problems, a history of seizures, or a shunt.

Vestibular stimulation can be organized to be either excitatory or inhibitory to the child's central nervous system. This is accomplished through movement control and combination. Movement into neck and body flexion (fetal position) tends to be organizing and focusing, while movements into neck and trunk extension tend to be arousing (Figure 6-9). Having the child organize a particular response to each movement tends to encourage a balance between the excitatory and inhibitory aspects of brain function.

Vestibular input calming activities follow principles similar to those associated with tactile input. The techniques are slow, steady, and rhythmic, relying on principles of organization and inhibition.

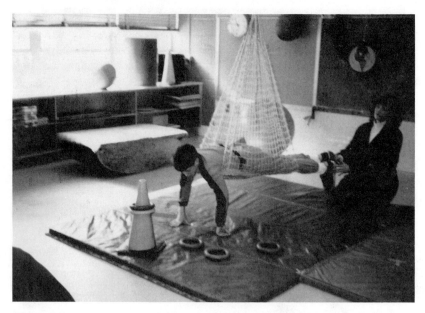

Figure 6-9. Working toward prone extension through movement.

The vestibular input is paired with proprioceptive, tactile, visual, and/or auditory input also designed to be calming. Inhibitory vestibular stimulation can be achieved by letting the child lie or sit securely on any comfortable suspended equipment and swinging him passively back and forth or in an orbit at a rate of 20 to 30 revolutions a minute. If suspended equipment is not an option because of fear, level of arousal, or availability, then the child may be rocked over a large therapy ball or bolster.

The fragile X child may have a variety of different reactions to vestibular input, depending on his level of neurological functioning, stress, and other experiences. If the child expresses fear or anxiety, then he will not be able to integrate the input and respond to it in an adaptive manner. The therapist needs to design a slow, safe approach to introduce and develop mastery of vestibular stimulation for the fearful or anxious child. If the child is gravitationally insecure, he will have an irrational fear of leaving an upright position, having his feet leave the ground, or being inverted. He may have behavioral or emotional concerns because of his total fear of movement. For this type of child, the movement activity should be carefully graded, prepared for, and paired with proprioceptive input applied downward to his head to facilitate improved processing of gravitational security.

The child with fragile X may seek out vestibular stimulation and initially demonstrate diminished activity, but will often quickly rebound and become overstimulated by the input. His responses should be watched carefully for interpretation and anticipation of the probable manner of input processing by his brain. Each movement should be paired with a purposeful outcome, to facilitate organization and increased processing. Movements that are too fast, lack purpose, or change too often in speed and/or direction tend to be overstimulating for the child with fragile X. Purposeful outcomes will involve planned, coordinated movements or language production (Chapter 8). These outcomes need to be paired with good auditory and/or visual attending skills to be fully integrating.

Visual

Basic Goals.   The therapist provides visual input to facilitate improved eye control in order to help the child improve eye contact, see lines, forms, and shapes correctly, see letters in reading, follow a line of print, and develop visual motor perceptions and eye hand coordination.

Goals for therapy include (Novakovich, 1989, p. 90):

- Indicate awareness of visual stimuli.
- Visually regard objects.
- Track moving objects.
- Demonstrate improved visual localization of objects.
- Demonstrate improved visual convergence.
- Focus on pertinent visual information in presence of competing stimuli.
- Decrease visual self-stimulation.

Other goals important to the child with fragile X include increased eye contact with people and improved visual perceptual and visual motor skills.

Principles and Techniques for Treatment.   Visual stimulation is controlled for size, shape, color, and distance, and is organized for calming, alerting, organizing, and processing purposes. Examples of designing calming visual input include using a natural low-light setting; use of large, uncluttered pictures and objects; and decreased extraneous visual input. The visual input should be presented slowly, one or two items at time and placed directly in front of the child's face, with time allowed for the youngster to visually adjust before moving it closer.

Visual alerting stimulation is used to increase the child's visual focus. Techniques include increasing the light intensity and colors and presenting the input quickly and at sporadic intervals. To increase the child's attention and focus, the therapist can use a flashlight; toys that blink, flash, or move; or blinking lights. Care should be taken to avoid overstimulation. These principles should be considered when selecting computer programs.

Visual stimulation requires a visual-motor or visual-perceptual task outcome to determine the effectiveness of the visual input. Visual perception and visual motor skills are facilitated by integrating activities with the sensory motor program. Treatment in this area includes eye-hand coordination, constructive spatial tasks, and visual perceptual tasks requiring higher cognitive function. Specific strategies are discussed later in this chapter.

Compensatory Strategies.   Compensatory skills for visual avoidance include having the child wear a hat or sunglasses to block some of the visual input. The therapist or teacher can make compensations to decrease visual stimulation intensity for the fragile X child by positioning herself so she is not directly in front of the child and by presenting any visual information to her side. In individual work, the teacher or therapist may even position herself behind the student. Classroom modifications include use of a carrel, covered shelves and supply areas, limited display of materials, and use of an overlay to block part of a page.

Auditory Input

Basic Goals. The therapist provides auditory input to enhance the child's ability to appropriately assimilate and use what he hears. This OT area can overlap with activities typically in the speech-language therapist's domain. Nevertheless, the OT will employ a variety of auditory inputs, including music, quiet noises for calming, and her voice as part of a multisensory approach to encourage adaptive responses from the child with fragile X. This is covered in more depth in Chapter 7.

Goals for the OT include (Novakovich, 1989, p. 74):

- Respond to auditory input.
- Localize source of sound.
- Focus on pertinent auditory stimuli in presence of competing stimuli.
- Discriminate auditory stimuli.

- Demonstrate improved recall of auditory stimuli.
- Demonstrate appropriate auditory attending behavior.
- Decrease auditory self-stimulation.

Gustatory Input

Basic Goals. The therapist provides gustatory or taste input in order to facilitate oral motor skill development for eating and speaking, increase tolerance for a variety of foods, and enhance sensory input that is effective in organizing and calming the central nervous system.

Goals for this area include (Novakovich, 1989, p. 74):

- React to taste input.
- Accept taste input.
- Discriminate foods with varying properties using taste.
- Decrease gustatory self-stimulation.

Other goals for fragile X children include introducing texture and improving oral motor control. These are examined closely in Chapter 7.

Principles and Techniques for Treatment. Oral input may be provided through touch or food presentation. Touch input to the external and internal oral structures is frequently used as a warm-up activity and to facilitate improved oral motor control. Food input can be grouped according to taste, texture, and temperature. Oral input can be organizing and/or stimulating. Examples of how to set up an oral stimulation program that is calming or organizing include rubbing lotion on the face; pressing the cheeks, chin, and lips firmly using touch-pressure; introducing warm food temperatures; and sucking activities using a variety of crazy straws, varying the thickness of the liquid to be sucked.

The oral stimulation program can arouse the child's nervous system through: quick, light pats to the child's face to increase muscle tone; crunchy, firm, and mixed textured foods to increase chewing and oral exploration of the food; cold, tart, and sweet taste experiences; and rubbing the inside of the mouth with a toothbrush to increase awareness and movements of the lips, tongue, and jaw. Activities causing further arousal to the fragile X child's nervous system are used to facilitate improved oral skills, but care should be taken not to pursue them to the point of overstimulation.

Compensatory Strategies.   Compensatory strategies for excessive oral self-stimulation, decreased awareness, and poor oral-motor skills include finding socially appropriate foods and textures for the child to chew on. Sugarless candies and gum can be given freely during therapy, with the child given extra touch-pressure and propriocep-tive input to his chin and jaw. The child may be allowed to use vibrators and electric toothbrushes as part of his oral play and exploration during therapy to accommodate his increased need for oral motor input. Visual, verbal, and tactile cues may be used to increase awareness and improve oral motor skills.

Olfactory

Basic Goals.   The therapist provides olfactory input to facilitate normalized processing of smell. Goals for this area include (Novakovich, 1989, p. 74):

- React to smell input.
- Tolerate smell input.
- Localize smell input.
- Identify substances or objects by smell.
- Decrease olfactory self-stimulation.

Principles and Techniques for Treatment.   Therapy techniques in-clude using natural odors and food smells, and avoiding strong, noxious smells. Therapy focuses on pairing and organizing the ol-factory input with other sensory input such as touch, taste, and vision. For example, the child may be asked to describe the smell of a food before he tastes it. Scented pens and stamp pads can be paired with verbal color labels. Olfactory stimulation generally has an alerting and organizing affect on the child's nervous system. The purposeful outcomes which are usually paired with smell input are cognitive and/or language tasks.

Phase Two: Sensory Processing

Body Scheme

At this phase of sensory integration, the child is sorting, organizing, combining, and processing information from all the senses to produce a response. Before a response can be accurate, the child must have a good blueprint of his body formed in his brain, telling him the relationship among his body parts and how they operate. Tactile, vestibular, visual, and proprioceptive input is combined and integrated to form the child's body scheme. Goals for improving a child's awareness of his body position and location in space focus first on oral-tactile exploration, then manipulation of materials with hands, before focusing on increased awareness of other body parts and their function. Once the child is aware of how his body moves and works effectively, he begins to be able to move according to commands, with a demonstrated awareness of how body parts relate to each other and to the environment. He can demonstrate awareness of the concepts of top/bottom, front/back, left/right, and other directional and positional words. The therapist helps the child through this developmental process by organizing the treatment environment and sensory information to be presented and guiding the child's sensory motor activities. The child must use self-directed play to gain a sense of self, explore his skill levels, and interact with the world around him to form a useful body scheme.

Figure-Ground

As information from any or all of the different senses is processed and organized, the brain screens out unnecessary input, thus allowing the child to better focus on the task at hand, plan what he is to do, and respond meaningfully. Intervention techniques for improved screening include use of a prescriptive environment, strategies for stress management, and sensory motor play. The prognosis for changing internal control of sensory input for a fragile X child is limited. This is not to say that behavior cannot be changed through appropriate intervention, however. The child may be taught compensatory strategies for dealing with his lack of ability to screen out unnecessary input, including appropriate self-stimulatory techniques to calm and organize himself and reduce stress, as well as to make changes to his environment so he can better cope with the world.

Praxis

Using information to regulate, monitor and plan for new motor skills is known as motor planning or praxis. Treatment that focuses on motor planning deals with the variety and quality of what the child plans, how he sequences his plan, and his execution of movement (Goodgold-Edwards & Cermak, 1989). Cues are used to facilitate use of proprioceptive feedback in learning by doing, effective timing mechanisms, and graded movement responses. Activities are graded from simple to complex by the number of steps involved and the level of difficulty of the task. Treatment employs suspended and gross motor equipment combined in challenging and innovative ways to form obstacle courses. Obstacle courses may be assembled completely by the therapist, or the child may help create the course. Either the therapist or the child formulates the plan for how to interact with the equipment, depending on the child's level of praxis skills. No matter what the goal, virtually every treatment activity that requires the child to plan and produce projected action sequences will facilitate motor planning (Figures 6-10 & 6-11). For the child with fragile X, who has significant sequencing problems, it will be important to gradually increase the number of steps or parts for him to examine in his plan. An important goal is to enable the child to approach novel sequential tasks with greater ease.

Foundations for Movement

Bilateral Integration.   The therapist is able to effect change in the child's movement patterns and improve his coordination through facilitation of bilateral integration, postural control, and postural security. Goals for bilateral integration focus on bringing hands and objects to the midline, crossing the midline, and using two hands

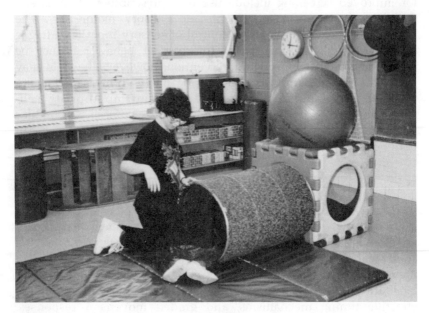

Figure 6-10. A motor-planning activity . . .

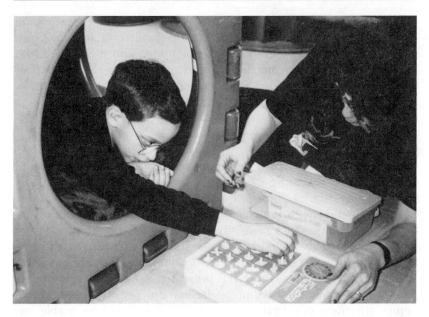

Figure 6-11. . . . results in an enclosed, non-distracting environment for performing a visual-motor task.

or feet in a coordinated, simultaneious manner. Bilateral movements can involve one extremity as a stabilizer and the other as a manipulator, or both extremities used either in parallel or opposing movements. The sequence of bilateral motor control development is from discrete to sequenced bilateral movements, and from symmetrical to alternating bilateral movements. Inhibition of associated reactions is critical for improved coordination for fragile X children.

Postural Control.   Goals for postural control include tone, cocontraction, body alignment, proximal stability, and balance. Goals for postural security include normalized movement patterns, balance, and movement against gravity. Chosen activities should encourage a variety of head positions to facilitate integration and maturation of primitive reflexes. The first focus in helping the child develop postural control is to assist him to assume and maintain prone extension through movement (Figure 6-9). Before working on the total body, resistance needs to be increased and extension challenged in the neck and upper back. Movement is most effective in a prone horizontal plane. Supine flexion is the next focus. Activities with resistance to movement into flexion are given, beginning with neck and abdominal muscles and working toward whole body patterns. Vertical stimulation devices and movement in a supine horizontal position are most effective for facilitating flexion. Once flexion and extension patterns can be assumed and maintained, the last focus is on combining flexion and extension into a variety of movement patterns needed for developing lateral flexion and trunk rotation. This leads to improved righting and equilibrium reactions.

Postural-Ocular Deficits

The goals for bilateral integration, postural control, and postural security, while sounding very different, share the requirement for improved vestibular and proprioceptive processing to facilitate changes. Goals seek to remediate postural ocular deficits, with ocular referring to compensatory eye movements initiated by the vestibular system in an attempt to maintain a stable visual field. Treatment techniques include use of NDT, sensory motor exploration, and use of functional activities. An NDT program addresses weight shifts and use of trunk rotation using facilitation. Sensory motor techniques stimulate vestibular and proprioceptive input to enable improved coordinated movements of the child's body and extremities and postural control during movements against gravity. A functional treatment approach utilizes activities of daily living (ADL) training, with a focus on improving skills through improved coordination of movement.

A by-product of sensory motor treatment not generally addressed in isolation is improvement of dissociation of eye movements from head and body. Ayres (1972) found a profound and positive influence on extra-ocular muscle control, without the use of overt eye exercises, in children who had learning disabilities. The results of this study form the foundation for treatment principles addressing ocular mechanisms. Sensory motor activities need to be chosen that challenge the child's ability to produce visually controlled ocular movements and separate head and eye movements for tracking and finding visual targets. The visual input provided during an activity should be controlled for speed, quantity, and duration of visual inspection and the organization of the materials. Referral to an optometrist or ophthalmologist may be warranted for further treatment.

A developmental optometrist should be sought if vision training activities or vision therapy services are desired. Vision therapy typically involves a series of treatments with carefully planned activities carried out by the patient under professional supervision to relieve visual problems. Vision therapy is not instituted to simply strengthen eye muscles, but rather is generally done to treat functional deficiencies for the patient to achieve optimal efficiency and comfort. Particular procedures and instruments are dependent on the nature of the visual dysfunction and the doctor's clinical judgment. Efficacy studies (Cohen, 1988) validate vision therapy as a therapeutic tool of remediation. The American Optometric Association affirms that vision therapy is an effective therapeutic modality in the treatment of many physiological and information processing dysfunctions of the vision system; however, further research is still needed on the subject (Cohen 1988; Livermore, 1988). At Ivymount School, vision therapy has been successful with fragile X children in conjunction with a comprehensive sensory motor program.

Phase Three: Cognitive and Motor Output

Now that the assimilation and processing of sensory information has been enhanced and a motor response developed, the foundations are in place for the next phase of treatment. This phase includes developing visual-spatial perception, auditory perception, and motor coordination. (Oral motor coordination and auditory-perceptual skill training are addressed in Chapter 7.) At this level, the brain coordinates information with body responses to determine how the child will interact with his environment. As the brain develops the capacity to perceive, integrate, remember, and motor plan, these abilities can be applied toward mastery of all learning as well as development of the conceptual abilities needed for the process of learning.

Cognitive Output

Visual-spatial perception includes form constancy, awareness of position in space, space visualization, figure-ground, and visual sequencing. Goals focus on the child being able to visually discriminate and understand the position of objects, pictures, and symbols in space, individually and in sequenced patterns. These lead to improved memory, organizational skills, and reading readiness. Sensory integration techniques address the sensory processing on which perceptual discriminations are based, and NDT techniques deal with proprioceptive and kinesthetic perceptions as they relate to functional movement patterns. These approaches provide training in the perceptual processing components of functional behavior with perceptual drills or specific sequences of sensory motor exercises (Neistadt, 1990). Perceptual motor treatment emphasizes the direct remediation of observed deficits through tabletop exercises, educational and functional activities, and practice drills. Activities are set up that control the environment or associated context, the familiarity, the directions given, the amount of objects present at one time, the spatial arrangement, and the response rate (Figure 6-11). However, care must be taken to address the underlying problem causing the dysfunction. For the child with fragile X, this is under- and overattention to detail, causing him to misperceive the whole. Treatment is on a continuum from simple to more complex activities, with reevaluation constantly conducted. Visual attention, assimilation, and decoding processes are evaluated through observation of performance and discussion with the child. Language deficits must also be ruled out as a factor interfering with object recognition and ability to understand and follow the directions given for the perceptual task. The therapist then uses a system of graded cues and investigative questioning to gain insight into the underlying reasons for a child's difficulty and facilitate changes in his processing. Toglia (1989) mentions that if the child's responses cannot be facilitated through cues or through task grading, then a treatment approach such as the cognitive rehabilitation method just outlined, which incorporates these tools, may not be the treatment of choice. In such a case, a sensory motor or functional approach might be more effective.

Motor Output

Principles of treatment for addressing coordination deficits, including eye-hand, in-hand manipulation, and whole-body movements follow developmental guidelines. The child's coordination skills develop proximally to distally, in a medial-lateral direction, from gross to refined movement patterns, and from a focus on stability to mobility. Development does not follow a linear path, but progresses in step-like stages or in spiraling patterns. For the child with fragile X, development of coordination is delayed or altered, because of his sensory integrative deficits and the associated lack of experience.

Therapeutic techniques for facilitating improved coordination involve the use of motor skill learning theories. Two different approaches to the facilitation of motor learning are presented. Information from both techniques is helpful in setting up a treatment program to improve the fragile X child's coordination. Gliner (1985) presents a treatment based on an event approach to motor skill acquisition. In his "Ecological Approach" to motor learning, he defines coordination as a relationship between the child and the environment, where neither is subordinate to the other.

Most important in this perspective is the notion that no skill can be conceived of without special reference to the immediate object; the environment must be included as the necessary support for coordinated, skilled movements. Therapeutic techniques focus on assisting the child with his processing of and adaptation to the environment. Gliner defines the variables involved in motor learning as being those variables specific to the environment and to the child. The problem for the learner is to discover a combination of the many variables, such as which joints are needed to carry out the child's intention, and limit these variables until further skill is acquired.

Janet Poole (1991) gives some valuable guidelines for the application of motor learning principles in occupational therapy. In her review of literature, she defines the four factors that influence motor learning as: (a) the stages of learning, (b) the type of task, (c) feedback, and (d) practice. The three sequential stages involved in the motor learning process are described as the cognitive stage, the associative stage, and the autonomous stage. In the cognitive stage, the child must try to understand the requirements of the motor task. Skills required at this level include the ability to verbalize the sequence, understand the positional factors of the situation, and attend to the relevant information related to the skill. The therapist can use verbal instruction, demonstration, or manual guidance to suggest the idea of movement to the child. During the next stage, the associative stage, the child begins to practice and refine his skills. The child must be able to learn through trial and error, and be able to adjust his subsequent movements based on learning by doing and appropriate predictions. This requires an effective feedback system. The autonomous stage comes after the child has acquired independent skill use.

Two of Poole's variables are especially important for the therapist to consider. *Feedback* may be intrinsic or extrinsic. Intrinsic feedback is defined as the inherent sensory information from receptors in the muscles, joints, and tendons, as well as receptors in the visual and auditory systems. It may occur during or after the movement. Extrinsic feedback is defined as the information from an external source that augments the intrinsic feedback. It may be a therapist's cue or a timer. The therapist can provide two types of extrinsic feedback: knowledge of performance and knowledge of results.

Practice can be defined in several ways. The order of the tasks practiced can remain the same (blocked practice) or differ (random practice). The conditions of the task may vary across trials or may remain the same. The amount of a skill practiced can range from a single component of the task to practicing the task in its entirety. The fragile X child, because of his simultaneous learning style, may have difficulty practicing only one element of a task at a time. How the skill is practiced will depend on the child's stage of learning, how effective his feedback system is, and the type of task. Remember that, with a child who has fragile X, perseveration and sensory overload will be an important factor in determining the amount of repetition and how the practice is set up.

Coordination Goals and Strategies

Goals for improving eye-hand coordination focus on developing and using appropriate grasp and release patterns with a variety of manipulatives, tools, and educational devices, such as the computer or calculator. The typical child's coordination develops as a result of knowledge about skilled activity developed through past experience and maturation. The experiences and maturation of the child with fragile X are affected by his sensory motor deficits and cognitive limitations, which in turn impact on the quality of his coordination. Treatment, therefore, involves task analysis of the fine motor and cognitive aspects of an activity. For example, before a child is ready to work on handwriting, he must practice in-hand manipulation of toys and small tools, coloring and scribbling, and multisensory experiences. When his cognitive skills reach the point where print is meaningful, letters can then be introduced based on past fine motor development. General treatment techniques for developing coordinated functional movement skills are addressed in such books as the Skill Starter Series by Marsha Dunn Klein (1982 a & b, 1983, 1987) (see resource list).

The therapist working with a child with fragile X needs to incorporate calming and organizing techniques into her treatment program. These techniques facilitate improved grading of movements, timing, and slowing the child down. It is difficult to focus on and improve fine motor, eye-hand coordination or in-hand manipulation skills with many children who have fragile X, because of their impulsivity, hyperreaction to stress, and levels of sensory overload. The therapist should set up a therapeutic environment, use preparatory sensory activities, and provide calming input throughout the activity. She should position herself so she is not directly in front of the child or making too much eye contact during the manipulation activities. It may be less stressful for the child with fragile X if the manipulation training activities are components of a purposeful, educational, or recreational activity rather than a contrived situation. Keep in mind that when working with a child with fragile X, teach tasks correctly and in full the first time to alleviate the child's difficulties with sequential learning and perseveration.

The areas of treatment in phase three should not be isolated from each other in the development of a comprehensive SI program. Murray, Cermak, and O'Brien (1990) discuss the relationship between perception, constructional abilities, and coordination in children. They conclude, as a result of their study, that clumsiness appears to be related to some aspects of visual-perceptual ability. One should not assume, however, that because a child is poorly coordinated that he will necessarily have problems in visual perception. They state that neither motor skill nor visual perception is a unitary ability, and certain aspects of visual perception may be more closely related to coordination and fine motor performance than others. Similarly, motor coordination and praxis are not synonymous. The authors conclude that the relationship between clumsiness, praxis, and visual-perceptual deficits needs further study. Furthermore, because of the intertwining nature of these deficit areas and the characteristics of the child with fragile X, coordination, praxis, and visual perception may be most easily remediated using a functional approach. This is done by choosing an art, cooking, high-interest educational, daily living, or prevocational task.

The functional outcome of treatment is that the occupational therapist will have impacted how the child deals with and interacts with his environment for academic learning, activities of daily living, improved behavior, social/emotional development, speech and language skills, and vocational skill training. The OT may need to specifically address the areas of daily living, recreational, and vocational skill training depending on the fragile X child's program and its effectiveness in training him (Figures 6-12 & 6-13). The child with fragile X may need a lot of planned carryover from the classroom and repetition of activities to improve his functional skill level. Many books and training programs on these specific topics are available to assist the occupational therapist (see resource list). In addition to specific skill training, the occupational therapist can structure functional situations so that the child must use the sensory motor information available in order to effectively plan and carry out functional living skills. These include planning, problem-solving skills, showing creativity, and making adjustments as needed. Consultation with other team members and incorporation of an OT program into the classroom may be required to coordinate the child's total development and enhance his learning program. Sensory integration principles and techniques may need to be

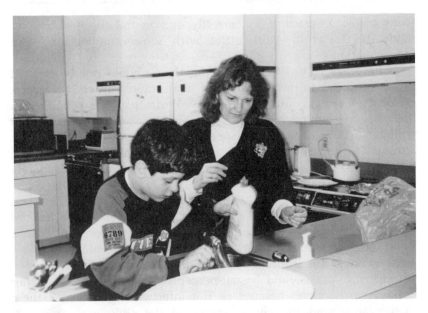

Figure 6-12. The occupational therapist works on activities of daily living.

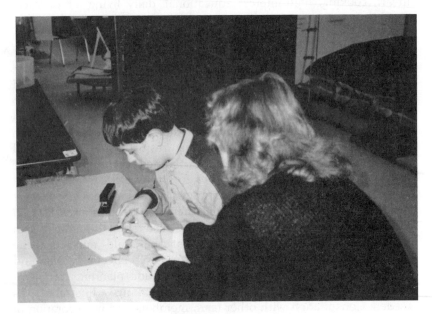

Figure 6-13. A pre-vocational activity.

permanently coordinated into the child's daily routine to compensate for his inadequate sensory processing caused by the fragile X. Lois Hickman has reported on the successful integration of a sensory integrative treatment approach into a summer camping experience for children with fragile X (Burns & Hickman, 1989), and into her treatment with adults who have fragile X (Hickman, 1990).

Treatment of Adults

Little is known about the use of a sensory integrative therapy program with adults. In an efficacy study regarding the use of sensory motor integrative treatment with mentally retarded adults, Huff and Harris (1987) were not able to find significant differences between their group of institutionalized subjects receiving treatment and their control group. However, because of the limitations imposed by institutionalization on vocational and other daily living skill training needs, there continues to be a potential role for the use of a sensory integrative approach in treatment of the adult with fragile X. Further research on the subject is needed. Lois Hickman (1990) suggests that consistent and frequent intervention is crucial in helping the adult with fragile X deal with frustration and to continue to acquire new skills. Appropriate calming techniques can be developed and practiced in therapy, and the adult can be taught how to incorporate the practices into his daily life (Scharfenaker & Hickman, 1989). We are providing services for the next generation of fragile X adults now. Because of increased knowledge of fragile X, this is perhaps the first generation of children with fragile X to be diagnosed early and provided with intensive treatment in more integrated mainstream settings. Their potential for growth, given early intervention with appropriate sensory integrative therapy, has yet to be fully determined. Their needs for SI as adults continue to be largely speculative. Goals for therapy must continue to focus on daily living activities and coping with the anxiety, stress, and frustrations associated with fragile X syndrome.

REFERENCES

American Occupational Therapy Association. (1979). Position statement defining occupational therapy. Rockville, AOTA, Inc.

American Occupational Therapy Association. (1986). Sensory integration information packet. Rockville, AOTA, Inc.

American Occupational Therapy Association. (1987). Setting priorities for providing services. In *Guidelines for occupational therapy services in school systems* (pp. 9.1-9.8). Rockville, AOTA, Inc.

Ayres, A.J. (1972). Improving academic scores through sensory integration. *Journal of Learning Disabilities, 5,* 23-28.

Ayres, A.J. (1973). *Sensory integration and learning disorders* (pp. 117, 119). Los Angeles: Western Psychological Services.

Ayres, A.J. (1975). *Southern California postrotary nystagmus test.* Los Angeles: Western Psychological Services.

Ayres, A.J. (1989). *Sensory integration and praxis test (SIPT).* Los Angeles: Western Psychological Services.

Berk, R., & Degangi, G. (1983). DeGangi-Berk test of sensory integration. Los Angeles: Western Psychological Services.

Blanche, E., & Burke, J. (1991a, March). Combining neuro-developmental and sensory integration approaches in the treatment of the neurologically impaired child. Part I. *Sensory Integration Quarterly, 19,* 1-5.

Blanche, E., & Burke, J. (1991b, June). Combining neuro-developmental and sensory integration approaches in the treatment of the neurologically impaired child. Part II. *Sensory Integration Quarterly, 19,* (1) 1-6.

Burns, E., & Hickman, L. (1989). Integrated therapy in a summer camping experience for children with fragile X syndrome. *Sensory Integration News, 17,* 1-3.

Cohen, A. (1988). The efficacy of optometric vision therapy. In 1986/87 future of visual development/performance task force. *Journal of the American Optometric Association, 59,* 95-105.

Devereaux, E. (1984). Occupational therapy's challenge: The caring relationship. *American Journal of Occupational Therapy, 38,* 791-798.

Dunn, W. (1981). A guide to testing clinical observations in kindergarteners. Rockville, MD: AOTA.

Farber, S., Scardina, V., & Lane, S. (1990, June). *Neuroscience institute: The sensory system.* American Occupational Therapy Association (conference), Baltimore, MD (handout).

Fisher, M.A. (1990). What is fragile X syndrome? Fragile X Association of Michigan, 1786 Edinborough Dr., Rochester Hills, MI, 48306.

Fisher, A., & Murray, E. (1991). Introduction to sensory integration theory. In A. Fisher, E. Murray, & A. Bundy (Eds.), *Sensory integration: Theory and practice* (pp. 1-27). Philadelphia: F.A. Davis Company.

Gliner, J. (1985). Purposeful activity in motor learning theory: An event approach to motor skill acquisition. *American Journal of Occupational Therapy, 39,* 28-36.

Goodgold-Edwards, S., & Cermak, S. (1990). Integrating motor control and motor learning concepts with neuropsychological perspectives on apraxia and developmental dyspraxia. *American Journal of Occupational Therapy, 44,* 431-440.

Grandin, T. (1988). Teaching tips from a recovered autistic. *Focus on Autistic Behavior, 3,* 1-8.

Haldy, M. (1987, December). A summer day camp experience for children with fragile X syndrome: A case study. *Sensory Integration Special Interest Section Newsletter, 10,* 2-3.

Hickman, L. (1988). Sensory integration and fragile X. *Fragile X Association of Michigan Newsletter, 6.*

Hickman, L. (1990, Fall/Winter). The challenges don't stop in childhood. *The National Fragile X Foundation Newsletter*, 2.

Huff, D., & Harris, S. (1987). Using sensorimotor integrative treatment with mentally retarded adults. *American Journal of Occupational Therapy, 41,* 227-231.

Jarek, K., & Bell, E. (1978). *Sensory integration at your finger tips.* Gonzales, TX: Texas Rehabilitation Hospital.

King-Thomas, L., & Hacker, B. (1987). *A therapist's guide to pediatric assessment.* Durham, NC: Developmental Therapy Association.

Klein, M.D. (1982a). *Pre-sign language motor skills.* Tuscon, AZ: Communication Skill Builders, Inc.

Klein, M.D. (1982b). *Pre-writing skills.* Tuscon, AZ: Communication Skill Builders, Inc.

Klein, M.D. (1983). *Pre-dressing skills.* Tuscon, AZ: Communication Skill Builders, Inc.

Klein, M.D. (1987). *Pre-scissor skills.* Tuscon, AZ: Communication Skill Builders, Inc.

Krauss, K. (1987). The effects of deep pressure touch on anxiety. *American Journal of Occupational Therapy, 41,* 366-373.

Livermore, B., (1988, August). Eyes in training: Is vision therapy oversold or underestimated? *Health,* 70-79.

Mailloux, Z. (1990). An overview of the sensory integration and praxis tests. *American Journal of Occupational Therapy, 44,* 589-594.

Murray, E., Cermak, S., & O'Brien, V. (1990). The relationship between form and space perception, constructional abilities, and clumsiness in children. *American Journal of Occupational Therapy, 44,* 623-629.

Neistadt, M. (1990). A critical analysis of occupational therapy approaches for perceptual deficits in adults with brain injury. *American Journal of Occupational Therapy, 44,* 299-305.

Novakovich, H. (Ed.). (1989). *Databased individual school curriculum (DISC).* Rockville, MD: The Ivymount School.

Poole, J. (1991). Application of motor learning principles in occupational therapy. *American Journal of Occupational Therapy, 45,* 531-538.

Royeen, C., & Fortune, J. (1990). Touch inventory for elementary school aged children. *American Journal of Occupational Therapy, 44,* 155-159.

Scardina, V. (1981). From pegboards to integration. *American Journal of Occupational Therapy, 35,* 581-588.

Scharfenaker, S., & Hickman. L. (1989, Spring). A combined approach to therapy with the fragile X adult. *The Fragile X Association of Michigan Newsletter,* 5-6.

Scharfenaker, S., Hickman L., & Braden M. (1991). An integrated approach to intervention. In R. Hagerman & A.C. Silverman (Eds.) *Fragile X syndrome: Diagnosis, treatment and research,* (pp. 327-372). Baltimore, MD: Johns Hopkins University Press.

Sensory Integration International. (1986). *A parent's guide to understanding sensory integration.* Torrance, CA: Sensory Integration International.

Toglia, J.P. (1989). Visual perception of objects: An approach to assessment and intervention. *American Journal of Occupational Therapy, 43,* 587-595.

Tutterow, J. (1988 Spring). Things to do at home (without becoming a therapist). *The National Fragile X Foundation Newsletter*, 5.

Van Hausen, K., (1987, Winter). Hypersenitivity and the fragile X child. *The National Fragile X Foundation Newsletter*, 2-3.

Wilbarger, P., & Royeen, C. (1987, November). *Tactile defensiveness: Theory, research and treatment of sensory affective disorders*. Rockville, MD (conference notes).

Wiss, T., & Clark, F. (1990). Validity of the Southern California postrotary nystagmus test: Misconceptions lead to incorrect conclusions. *American Journal of Occupational Therapy, 44*, 658-660.

ADDITIONAL READINGS—EFFICACY OF SENSORY INTEGRATION

Angelo, J.K.B. (1980). Effects of sensory integration treatment on the low-achieving college student. *American Journal of Occupational Therapy, 34*, 671-675.

Arendt, R.E., MacLean, W.E., & Baumeister, A. (1988). Critique of sensory integration therapy and its application in mental retardation. *American Journal on Mental Retardation, 92*, 401-411.

Arnold, L., Clark, D., Sachs, L., Jakim, S., & Smithics, C. (1985). Vestibular and visual rotational stimulation as treatment for attention deficits and hyperactivity. *American Journal of Occupational Therapy, 39*, 84-91.

Ayres, A.J. (1972). Improving academic scores through sensory integration. *Journal of Learning Disabilities, 5*, 24-28.

Ayres, A.J. (1978). Learning disabilities and the vestibular system. *Journal of Learning Disabilities, 11*, 30-41.

Ayres, A.J., & Mailloux, Z. (1981). Influence of sensory integration procedures on language development. *American Journal of Occupational Therapy, 35*, 383-390.

Ayres, A.J., & Tickle, L.S. (1980). Hyper response to touch and vestibular stimulation as a predictor of positive response to sensory integration procedures by autistic children. *American Journal of Occupational Therapy, 34*, 375-381.

Bhatara, V., Clark, D.L., & Arnold, L.E. (1978). Behavioral and nystagmus response of a hyperkinetic child to vestibular stimulation. *American Journal of Occupational Therapy, 32*, 311-316.

Bhatara, V., Clark, D.L., Arnold, L.E., Gunsett, R., & Smeltzer, D.J. (1981). Hyperkinesis treated by vestibular stimulation: An exploratory study. *Biology and Psychiatry, 16*, 269-279.

Bonadonna, P. (1981). Effects of a vestibular stimulation program on stereotypic rocking behavior. *American Journal of Occupational Therapy, 35*, 775-781.

Bright, T., Bittick, K., & Fleeman, B. (1981). Reduction of self-injurious behavior using sensory integrative techniques. *American Journal of Occupational Therapy, 35*, 167-172.

Carto, E., Drake, W.E., & Morrison, D.C. (1983). *CHILD center study on the effects of sensory integration therapy on the functioning of learning handicapped children* (Project summary). Kentfield, CA: Childhood Help in Learning and Development.

Cermak, S., & Henderson, A. (1990). The efficacy of sensory integration procedures: Part I. *Sensory Integration Quarterly, 17,* 1-5.

Cermak, S., & Henderson, A. (1990). The efficacy of sensory integration procedures: Part II. *Sensory Integration Quarterly, 18,* 1-4.

Clark, D.L., Kreutzberg, J.R., & Chee, F.K.W. (1977). Vestibular stimulation influence on motor development in infants. *Science, 196,* 1228-1229.

Clark, F.A., Miller, L.R., Thomas, J.A., Kucherawy, D.A., & Azen, S.P. (1978). A comparison of operant and sensory integrative methods on developmental parameters in profoundly retarded adults. *American Journal of Occupational Therapy, 32,* 86-92.

Clark, F., & Pierce, D. (1988). Synopsis of pediatric occupational therapy effectiveness: Studies on sensory integrative procedures, controlled vestibular stimulation, other sensory stimulation approaches, and perceptual motor training. *Sensory Integration News, 16,* 1-15.

Danner, P., & Clark, F. (1983). *Effectiveness of sensory integration procedures on four Finnish preschoolers with minimal brain dysfunction.* Unpublished master's thesis, University of Southern California Los Angeles.

Fisher, A., & Dunn, W. (1983). Tactile defensiveness: Historical perspectives, new research — A theory grows. *Sensory Integration Special Interest Section Newsletter, 6,* 1-3.

Grimwood, L.M., & Rutherford, E.M. (1980). Sensory integrative therapy as an intervention procedure with grade one "at risk" readers—a three year study. *The Exceptional Child, 27,* 52-61.

Kantner, R.M., Kantner, B., & Clark, D.L. (1982). Vestibular stimulation effect on language development in mentally retarded children. *American Journal of Occupational Therapy, 36,* 36-41.

MacLean, W.E., & Baumeister, A.A. (1982). Effects of vestibular stimulation on motor development and stereotyped behavior of developmentally delayed children. *Journal of Abnormal Child Psychology, 10,* 229-245.

Magrun, W.M., Ottenbacher, K., McCue, S., & Keefe, R. (1981). Effects of vestibular stimulation on spontaneous use of verbal language in developmentally delayed children. *American Journal of Occupational Therapy, 35,* 101-104.

Montgomery, P., & Richter, E. (1977). Effect of sensory integrative therapy on the neuromotor development of retarded children. *Journal of the American Physical Therapy Association, 57,* 799-806.

Oetter, P. (1986, June). A sensory integrative approach to the treatment of attention deficit disorders. *Sensory Integration Newsletter, 19,* 1-2.

Ostrow, P., Lawlor, M., & Joe, B. (1988). Research supports efficacy of sensory integration procedures. *Efficacy Data Brief, 3,* 1-6.

Ottenbacher, K. (1982). Sensory integration therapy: Affect or effect? *American Journal of Occupational Therapy, 36,* 571-578.

Ottenbacher, K. (1991). Research in sensory integration: Empirical perceptions and progress. In A.G. Fisher, E.A. Murray, & A.C. Bundy

(Eds.), *Sensory Integration: Theory and practice* (pp. 385-401). Philadelphia: F.A. Davis Company.

Ray, T., King, L.J., & Grandin, T. (1988). The effectiveness of self-initiated vestibular stimulation in producing speech sounds in an autistic child. *The Occupational Therapy Journal of Research, 8,* 187-190.

Resman, M.H. (1981). Effects of sensory stimulation on eye contact in a profoundly retarded adult. *American Journal of Occupational Therapy, 35,* 31-35.

Tickle-Degnen, L. (1988). Perspectives on the status of sensory integration theory. *American Journal of Occupational Therapy, 42,* 427-433.

Urbanik, C. (1986, March). Sensory integrative treatment for people with developmental disabilities. *Developmental Disabilities Newsletter, 9,* 1-2.

Weeks, Z. (1979a). Effects of the vestibular system on human development, part 1: Overview of functions and effects of stimulation. *American Journal of Occupational Therapy, 33,* 376-381.

Weeks, Z. (1979b). Effects of the vestibular system on human development, part 2: Effects of vestibular stimulation on mentally retarded, emotionally disturbed, and learning disabled individuals. *American Journal of Occupational Therapy, 33,* 450-457.

White, M. (1979). A first-grade intervention program for children at risk for reading failure. *Journal of Learning Disabilities, 12,* 26-32.

ADDITIONAL READINGS— OCCUPATIONAL THERAPY

Sensory Motor

Ayres, A.J. (1979). Sensory integration and the child. Los Angeles: Western Psychological Services.

Baker, B., Brightman, A., & Blacher, J. (1983). *Play skills.* Champaign, IL: Research Press.

Bissell, J., Fisher, J., Owens, C., & Pokyn, P. (1988). *Sensory motor handbook: A guide for implementing and modifying activities in the classroom.* Torrance, CA: Sensory Integration International Publishers.

Boehme, R. (1988). *Improving upper body control: An approach to assessment and treatment of tonal dysfunction.* Tucson, AZ: Therapy Skill Builders.

Brandreth, G. (1981). *The world's best indoor games.* New York: Pantheon Books.

Clark, P., & Allen, A. (1985). *Occupational therapy for children.* St. Louis, MO: C.V. Mosby Company.

Click, M., & Davis, J. (1982). *Moving right along.* Mesa, AZ: EdCorp.

Connolly, B., & Montgomery, P. (1987). *Therapeutic exercise in developmental disabilities.* Chattanooga, TN: Chattanooga Corporation.

Farber, S. (1989). Neuroscience and occupational therapy: Vital connections. *American Journal of Occupational Therapy, 43,* 637-646.

Feretti (1975). *The great American book of sidewalk, stoop, dirt, curb, and alley games.* New York: Workman Publishing Company.

Folio, M.R., & Fewell, R. (1983). *Peabody developmental motor scales and activity cards.* Allen, TX: DLM Teaching Resources.

Kohl, M.A.F. (1989). *Mudworks: Creative clay, dough, and modeling experiences.* Bellingham, WA: Bright Ring Publishing.

Marzollo, J., & Lloyd, J. (1972). *Learning through play.* New York: Harper & Row.

Orlick, T. (1978). *The cooperative sports and games book: Challenge without competition.* New York: Pantheon Books.

Quirk, N., & DiMatties, M. (1990). *The relationship of learning problems and classroom performance to sensory integration.* Cherry Hill, NJ: Quirk and DiMatties.

Walker, K. (1991, Spring). Sensory integrative therapy in a limited space: An adaptation of the Ayres clinic design. *Sensory Integration Special Interest Section Newsletter, 14,* 1-5.

Young, S. (1988). *Movement is fun: A preschool movement program.* Torrance, CA: Sensory Integration International Publishers.

Fine Motor

Johnson-Levine, K. (1991). *Fine motor dysfunction: Therapeutic strategies in the classroom.* Tucson, AZ: Therapy Skill Builders.

Klein, M.D. (1982). *Pre-sign language motor skills.* Tuscon, AZ: Communication Skill Builders, Inc.

Klein, M.D. (1982). *Pre-writing skills.* Tuscon, AZ: Communication Skill Builders, Inc.

Klein, M.D. (1983). *Pre-dressing skills.* Tuscon, AZ: Communication Skill Builders, Inc.

Klein, M.D. (1987). *Pre-scissor skills.* Tuscon, AZ: Communication Skill Builders, Inc.

Sahlin-Siegling, L., & Click, M. (1984). *At arm's length: Goals for arm and hand function.* Mesa, AZ: EdCorp.

Daily Living

Baker, B., & Brightman, S. (1980). *Toward independent living.* Champaign, IL: Research Press.

Cooper, T., & Ratner, M. (1974). *Many hands cooking: An international cookbook for girls and boys.* New York: Thomas V. Crowell company in cooperation with the U.S. Committee for UNICEF.

Cox, B. (1979). *I can do it! I can do it! Cookbook for people with very special needs.* Newport Beach, CA: Kitt Publishing Company.

Cox, B. (1981). *I can do it! I can do it! Housekeeping hints for people with very special needs.* Newport Beach, CA: Kitt Publishing Company.

Doyle, E., & Beam, J. (1983). *Daily experiences and activities for living housing.* Allen, TX: Developmental Learning Materials.

Evans-Morris, S., & Dunn-Klein, M. (1987). *Pre-feeding skills: A comprehensive resource for feeding development.* Tucson, AZ: Therapy Skill Builders.

Merrick, L., Schopmeyer, B., & Kaye, S. (1988). *Skills for independent living: A curriculum framework.* Rockville, MD: Ivymount School.

Orelove, F., & Sobsey (1987). *Educating children with multiple disabilities: A transdisciplinary approach.* Baltimore, Paul H. Brookes.

Sudol, E. (1985). *Look'n cook: Cookbook and curriculum guide.* Oregon, WI: Attainment Company Education and Training Materials.

Wilcox, B., & Bellamy, G.T. (1987). *The activities catalog: An alternative curriculum for youth and adults with severe disabilities.* Baltimore, MD: Paul H. Brookes Publishing Company.

Vocational

Kirkland, M., & Robertson, S. (1985). *PIVOT: Planning and implementing vocational readiness in occupational therapy.* Rockville, American Occupational Therapy Association, Inc.

Sarkees, M.D., & Scott, J.L. (1986). *Vocational special needs.* Homewood, IL: American Technical Publishers, Inc.

RESOURCES—EQUIPMENT

SI Equipment Sources
Southpaw Enterprises
800 W. Third St.
Dayton, OH 45407.

Flaghouse, Inc.
18 W. 18th St.
New York, NY 10011

Preston Corporation
60 Page Rd.
Clifton, NJ 07012

Functional Equipment
Fred Sammons
145 Tower Dr.
Burr Ridge, IL 60521

7

SPEECH AND LANGUAGE THERAPY WITH THE FRAGILE X CHILD

The child with fragile X demonstrates a unique profile of speech and language deficits which must be addressed in speech and language therapy. The speech-language pathologist should be aware of the behaviors that are most characteristic of this population and the impact these behaviors have on treatment (Chapter 5). Speech and language intervention must consider a number of factors, including modifying the environment for the fragile X child, treating behaviors which interfere with learning, and treating the high level of anxiety demonstrated by fragile X boys—particularly when they have to deal with changes in their environment, transitions, greeting unfamiliar people, and learning new information. Hyperactivity and hyperreactivity (extreme sensitivity to stimuli) are also behaviors impacting on treatment.

AN INTEGRATED APPROACH

The fragile X child exhibits a vast array of speech and language, sensory processing, social-emotional, learning, and cognitive deficits that may be confusing and overlapping. In our experience, a team approach, with integrated educational, therapeutic, and medical services, is extremely important. This team should include the special education teacher, speech-language pathologist (SLP), occupational therapist (OT), physical therapist (PT), psychologist, social worker, physician, and parents. Service integration involves interaction among pertinent team members for a better understanding of the child's strengths and needs. Integration may also involve consultative or direct co-treatment between two or more related services. Combined treatment (Chapter 8) focuses on service integration involving the SLP and OT. Joint programming between the SLP and special education teacher is fostered when the SLP works in the classroom. The SLP and the social worker can target social language and social emotional skills in joint treatment. A multidisciplinary approach to intervention provides an integrated framework within which a child's educational programming can develop.

Service Delivery

There are a variety of models for delivering speech and language services to the fragile X child. The model chosen may be determined by the goals for the therapy session, the child's sensory needs for that day, and the services available in the educational setting.

Speech and language therapy can be delivered individually, or in small and large groups. Joint treatment is an alternative treatment model that can also be delivered individually or in groups. Boys with fragile X may perform better in group activities because the pressure to perform is decreased. Group therapy also allows the child to observe his peers modeling a targeted behavior. Choice of peers is also important when grouping the fragile X child. Consider choosing a peer who is low-keyed and calm and who will not add distractions or increase the activity level in the session.

The SLP provides treatment in a therapy room or other locations within or outside the school environment. While the traditional pull-out model has the advantage of limiting distracting input, language use is not as natural and meaningful in a therapy room as in other settings (playground, OT room, classroom, or outside of school). The scheduling of speech and language therapy may also be a factor in the delivery model. For example, the child with fragile X may benefit from receiving occupational therapy immediately before a speech and language session.

Assessment

A complete evaluation of the fragile X child's speech and language skills is needed before developing a treatment plan. An audiological evaluation should be performed to rule out the possibility of hearing loss or otitis media, which is frequently seen in the fragile X population (Chapter 5). Speech and language behaviors should be measured and described, using standardized tests and observation. A language evaluation should include assessment of: receptive and expressive vocabulary, expressive language organization, comprehension of lengthy and complex information, and pragmatic skills. Table 7-1 reviews the language skills that should be assessed and lists suggested formal and informal measures to evaluate each area. Schopmeyer and Pellegrino (Table 7-1) divide tests into categories reflecting the child's age and cognitive level. Formal testing should be conducted in an environment that limits distractions, reduces anxiety, and assists the child in remaining calm. For example, testing may be done in the OT room using therapeutic equipment. Calming techniques discussed in Chapter 6 may be used before and during testing, with documentation of strategies used to be annotated on the test form and in the written report. The child's anxiety may also be decreased by use of humor.

In addition to a language assessment, speech assessment should include: observation of the oral structures, imitation of oral movement, diadokinetic rate determination, a formal articulation test, a spontaneous speech sample, observation of the child while eating, and a feeding evaluation.

Goal Development

After completing an evaluation and determining the child's strengths and weaknesses, a treatment plan should be developed. Long-term goals that may be part of the fragile X child's Individual Education Plan (IEP) include: oral-motor control, intelligibility, vocabulary, auditory processing (attention, memory, and comprehension), syntax skills, expressive language organization, pragmatic (social) language ability, and critical thinking skills. The goals listed below are taken from the Databased Individual School Curriculum (DISC) manual from the Ivymount School (Novakovich, 1989, pp. 29-40) and are used to develop an IEP.

- Student will demonstrate improved oral-motor control for eating and speech.
- Student will demonstrate improved intelligibility (articulation, voice, fluency, rate, motor planning) in order to be understood by teachers and peers.

TABLE 7-1. Discriminative Tests: Fragile X Children. J. Pelligrino and B. Schopmeyer.

AREA	LOW LEVEL	MID LEVEL	HIGH LEVEL
Receptive Vocabulary	Peabody Picture Vocabulary Test (PPVT).[1]	PPVT.	PPVT.
	Receptive One-Word Picture Vocabulary Test (ROWPVT).[2]	ROWPVT.	ROWPVT. ROWPVT Upper Extension.[3]
Receptive Syntax	Test for Auditory Comprehension of Language— (rev. ed.) (TACL-R).[4]	TACL-R Test of Language Development— Primary (TOLD-P):[5] Grammatic Understanding.	TACL-R TOLD-P: Grammatic Understanding.
Following Directions	Preschool Language Scale:[6] direction items. Sequenced Inventory of Communication Development (SICD):[7] direction items.	Assessment of Children's Language Comprehension (ACLC).[8]	Token Test for Children.[9] Clinical Evaluation of Language Function (CELF-2):[10] Oral directions.
Concepts	SICD. Vocabaluary Comprehension Scale.[11]	Bracken Basic Concepts Scale.[12]	Bracken Basic Concepts Scale.
Expressive Vocabulary	Expressive One-Word Picture Vocabulary Test (EOWPVT).[13]	EOWPVT.	EOWPVT. EOWPVT Upper Extension[14]
Sentence Formulation and Organization	Preschool Language Assessment Inventory (PLAI).[15] Illinois Test of Psycholinguistic Abilities (ITPA):[16] Verbal Expression. Language Sample.	CELF: Formulated Sentences. Evaluating Communicative Competence:[17] Expressive Tasks. Language Sample.	Detroit Test of Learning Aptitude-2[18] (DTLA-2): Story Construction. Language Sample.

(continued)

TABLE 7-1.   *(continued)*

Expressive Syntax	ITPA: Grammatic Closure, Language Sample.	ITPA: Grammatic Closure. TOLD-P: Grammatic Completion. Language Sample.	TOLD-P: Grammatic Completion, Language Sample.
Sentence Repetition	PLAI: Sentence repetition items.	TOLD-P: Sentence imitation.	DTLA-2: Sentence imitation.
Social Language	Ivymount Pragmatic Skills Checklist. PLAI.	Ivymount Pragmatic Skills Checklist. Test of Pragmatic Skills.[19]	Ivymount Pragmatic Skills Checklist. Test of Pragmatic Skills.
Abstract Thinking	PLAI.	CELF: Semantic relationships.	Test of Problem Solving (TOPS).[20]

1. Dunn, L.M., & Dunn, L.M. (1981)
2. Gardner, M.F. (1985)
3. Brownell, R. (1987)
4. Carrow-Woolfolk, E. (1985)
5. Newcomer, P.L., & Hammill, D.D. (1988)
6. Zimmerman, I.L., Steiner, V.G., & Pond, R.E. (1979)
7. Hedrick, D.L., Prather, E.M., & Tobin, A.R. (1984)
8. Foster, R., Giddan, J.J., & Stark, J. (1973)
9. DiSimoni, F., (1978)
10. Semel, E., Wiig, E., Secord, W., & Sabers, D. (1987)
11. Bangs, T.E. (1975)
12. Bracken, B.A. (1984)
13. Gardner, M.F. (1979)
14. Gardner, M.F. (1983)
15. Blank, M., Rose, S.A., & Berlin, L.J. (1978)
16. Kirk, S.A. & Kirk, W.D. (1968)
17. Simon, C.S. (1984)
18. Hamill, D.D. (1985)
19. Shulman, B.B. (1986)
20. Zachman, I., Jorgensen, C., Hiusingh, R., & Barrett, M. (1984)

- Student will demonstrate knowledge of a more age-appropriate vocabulary in order to understand instruction and be able to respond more appropriately.

- Student will demonstrate comprehension of targeted auditory information in order to understand instructions, follow directions, and improve reading and math skills.

- Student will demonstrate improved social use of language in order to function more appropriately in school, at home, and in the community.
- Student will organize and express a message in order to communicate more effectively with teachers and peers.
- Student will demonstrate knowledge of targeted relationships in order to improve critical thinking skills and reasoning ability.
- Student will demonstrate ability to utilize an augmentative communication system in order to function in an educational setting.

The IEP also describes the frequency and delivery of services, the strategies for teaching these goals, and the criteria used to assess goal mastery. Short-term objectives are developed that describe specific steps leading to mastery of the long-term goals.

The remainder of this chapter is devoted to specific objectives and the strategies to help the fragile X child master them. Strategies are presented for use with preschool and school-aged fragile X boys who are learning disabled, or mild-to-moderately mentally retarded. Many of the methods discussed in this chapter are based on a review of the literature on learning disabilities, attention deficit disorder, apraxia, and mental retardation, plus consultation with therapists and teachers at the Ivymount School.

ORAL SENSORY MOTOR INTERVENTION

Boys with fragile X syndrome can be described as having deficits in the area of oral-motor skills. The therapist must have a strong knowledge of the anatomy and physiology of the oral musculature, as well as the normal development of oral-motor and feeding skills. This background knowledge is critical for understanding which aspects of the oral sensory motor and feeding profile of the fragile X child are normal, delayed, or deviant (Morris, 1985a). A remediation program must incorporate a combination of oral stimulation and feeding therapy to "normalize" the response to sensory input and improve motor function. Oral stimulation must address the normalization of movement and the functional use of the oral structures, including the jaw, cheeks, lips, tongue, and teeth. The following sections describe techniques to increase muscle tone and facilitate normal motor patterns. Many techniques have been pulled from the work of Suzanne Evans Morris (1977, 1985a, 1985b, 1987) and from workshops and inservice presentations on Neurodevelopmental Treatment (NDT) approach developed by Bobath (1987) for children with cerebral palsy.

Feeding therapy for children with fragile X focuses on improving nutrition, oral-sensory motor skills, plus the impact of eating skills on socialization. All of these skills require a joint effort by the SLP and the OT.

Goals for oral motor control include (Novakovich, 1989, pp. 29-30):

- Normalize sensitivity to tactile stimulation in the oral area;
- Demonstrate improved posture to support eating and speech;
- Improve muscle tone for eating and speech;
- Demonstrate adequate tongue, lip, and jaw movements for eating and speech;
- Demonstrate increased awareness of drooling.

Therapy Strategies: Physical Environment

The physical features of the therapy environment impact on the child's oral motor and eating skills. When developing a therapy program, consider seating and positioning for postural stability, movement and physical handling, use of food, structure and behavior modification, and individual vs. group therapy.

Seating and Positioning

Oral stability and mobility are dependent on neck and trunk stability and control. Optimum trunk stability depends on correct seating and positioning. There are a variety of positions which can successfully support the fragile X child's postural stability during oral motor and feeding therapy. When seating the child at a desk or table, the correct chair height must be determined, with the child's feet flat on the floor and a 90° angle at the ankles, knees, and hips (Figures 7-1 & 7-2). A younger child may sit on the therapist's lap for greater stability at the hips and to allow the therapist easier access to the oral musculature. Seating the child backwards on a chair, with forearms supported on the chair back, provides greater support to the upper body and decreases flexion (slumping over table). A therapy ball or hippity hop may be used for seating to challenge the child's balance and for trunk stability (Figure 7-3).

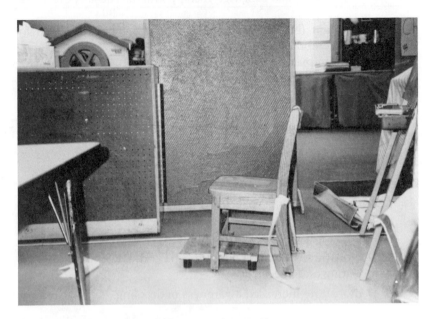

Figure 7-1. Chair adapted for appropriate seating.

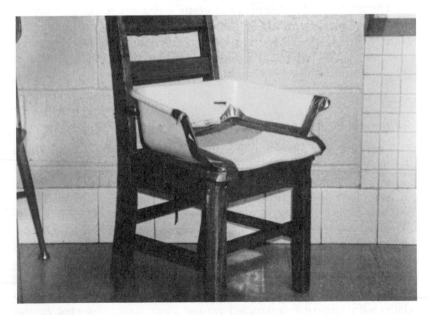

Figure 7-2. Chair adapted for appropriate seating.

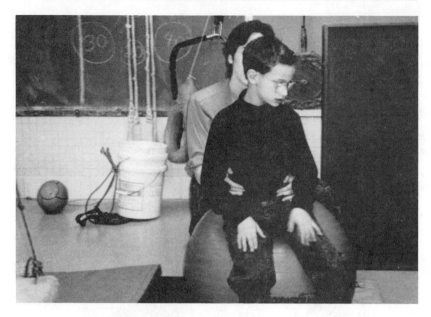

Figure 7-3. Child seated on therapy ball.

Physical Handling and Movement

Boys with fragile X often exhibit poor postural stability, decreased muscle tone, and poor motor planning that interfere with oral-motor and eating skills. Physical handling, oral-motor stimulation, and fine and gross motor exercises improve postural stability, increase muscle tone, and provide support for normal oral-motor patterns.

When planning gross and fine motor activities, consider beginning with distal areas, then working to proximal areas. Gross motor exercises should be introduced before fine motor. The gross motor activities will help to increase trunk stability and allow for greater mobility of fine motor movements of the oral musculature necessary for eating and speech. Stamping, galloping, jumping, and running are all activities which involve the whole body. They activate a variety of muscles and provide deep proprioceptive input that serves to increase muscle tone. Chair and wall push-ups, and hand-to-hand input provide proprioceptive input to the muscles and joints of the upper body (Figure 7-4 & 7-5). Other activities which increase tone include:

- Wheelbarrow walking;
- Placing child on stomach over a barrel so he must catch himself on his hands;

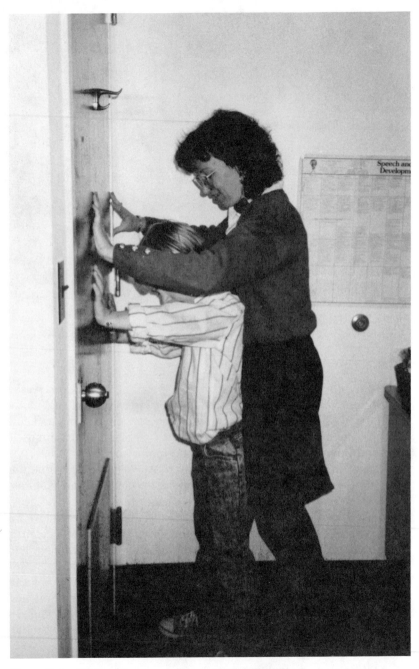

Figure 7-4. Wall push-ups provide proprioceptive input.

148

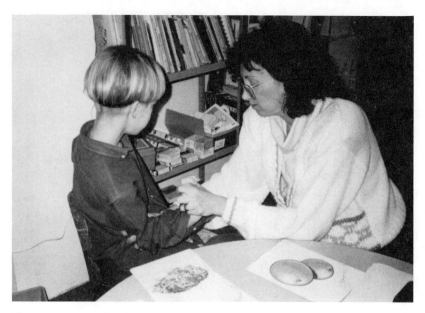

Figure 7-5. Hand to hand input.

- Placing child on his stomach on a wedge using his hands and arms to support his upper body (Figure 7-6);
- Therapist applying pressure to child's head, shoulders, and arms.

When physically handling the fragile X child, consider the type of touch and the direction of movement. Firm or deep pressure provides proprioceptive input for increased muscle tone. Light touch should be used for facilitation of movement so that the child has greater control, while the therapist guides the movement. Children with fragile X, however, may have difficulty tolerating light touch, and may require preparation using firm or deep pressure. The therapist must continually observe the child's response to these intrusive activities in order to assess their effectiveness and to be aware of the child's emotional response to the physical handling. The action of the movement should follow the direction of the muscle. For example, the buccinator muscle, which is the principle muscle of the cheeks, courses horizontally forward to the upper and lower lips. Movement should follow this direction.

To increase muscle tone and improve mobility of the tongue, lips, and cheeks, a variety of stimulation techniques may be used. Quick tapping, vibration, or deep pressure to these structures in-

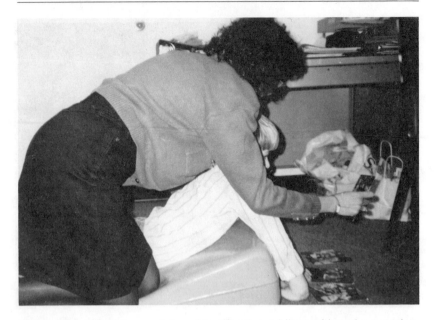

Figure 7-6. Working on picture identification while positioned on wedge.

creases tone. Deep stroking down the cheeks to the mouth alternating with quick tapping helps to improve lip closure, as does tapping and rubbing up on the bottom lip. Lipstick or chapstick provides proprioceptive input for lip closure. Making lipstick prints provides a visual cue for gradation of lip opening and is motivating to the child. Tone and mobility can also be addressed by brushing the tongue, gums, and teeth with a toothbrush (Figure 7-7), by placing a finger firmly on the front of the tongue, or with finger walking from the front to the back of the tongue. Some children are very hypersensitive on the tongue and may gag during these activities. Closing the jaw immediately after stimulation may prevent the child from gagging.

Physical Handling for Feeding

Parents of boys with fragile X often describe their children as messy eaters. Behaviors mentioned include: gags on food, doesn't like to try new foods, stuffs food, and plays with food. The SLP should include a feeding evaluation to determine if these behaviors are a function of delayed development, deviant motor patterns, a sensory processing deficit, or a combination. Since most boys with fragile X exhibit difficulties with sensory processing, many of these

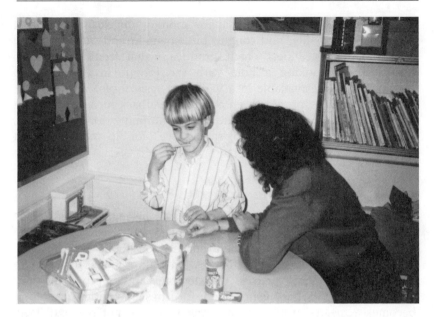

Figure 7-7. Oral-motor stimulation.

feeding issues will be sensory based. These are discussed in the section Sensory Environment. This section addresses issues related to motor deficits.

Observation of the oral structures should include an assessment of jaw stability, gradation of jaw opening when eating, rotary jaw movement during eating, separation of movement, lip closure when eating and drinking, tongue lateralization, and tongue elevation. When jaw stability and gradation is an issue, the therapist can assist jaw movement by cradling the chin between two fingers with the thumb placed by the jaw. To assist lip stability, place the index finger under the bottom lip and the thumb under the child's chin. This provides a stable surface for a cup. To stimulate movement in the upper lip, press down on the child's tongue with a spoon. This will stimulate the upper lip to clean off food. To improve tongue lateralization and tongue tip elevation, sweep or brush up on the lateral borders of the tongue and the tongue tip (Morris, 1977).

Physical Handling for Volitional Movement

A common motor deficit seen in boys with fragile X is dyspraxia, or difficulty with volitional movement. Movement that results in an auditory or visual feedback may assist in improving control. Use of a mirror will help the child visually monitor lip closure, size and shape of lip opening, and tongue placement in and outside of the mouth. Other activities which produce visual feedback include: lipstick prints, poking a hole with the tongue in theroplast (a therapeutic putty available in a variety of resistances), and blowing bubbles. Activities providing an auditory feedback include: growling to produce elevation of tongue back, humming for lip closure, squirrel talk using tongue tip, saying "ee" for lip retraction, and saying "u" for lip rounding.

Food

Specific goals for the fragile X child can be met by using foods to achieve a desired motor response or offer new sensory input. The section on Sensory Environment focuses on foods that provide sensory input. This section focuses on using foods to improve volitional movement, increase muscle tone, and improve mobility and placement. When using food for these activities, the food becomes a means to an end or target behavior, not the end itself. We often explain to the children that we will be doing some fun activities with food that we only do during SOM-G (sensory oral motor group). We do not copy these activities at mealtimes. SOM-G activities occur at a separate time and place from snack or lunch to reinforce the difference.

Tongue mobility can be targeted by using a lollipop to encourage in-out movement or by spreading a creamy food (e.g., peanut butter) on lips for a sweeping tongue action. Tongue placement can be targeted by placing peanut butter or honey on the corners of the lips for laterality, or on the alveolar ridge for elevation. Food can also be placed between the cheeks and lips for tongue laterality or by moving a small round lollipop from cheek to cheek. Lip rounding can be targeted by blowing or sucking liquid through a straw, or by sucking salt off a pretzel log.

Structure and Behavior Modification

Children with fragile X perform best in a highly structured learning environment. While this section focuses on adding structure to oral-motor and feeding therapy, use of structure should be incorporated into all therapy goals. A structured environment will help decrease the fragile X child's anxiety by providing him with known expectations and consequences. The child may learn that a therapy session begins with gross motor activities and follows with oral-motor stimulation or that activities are initially easy and become increasingly more challenging. This structure builds in repetition over time—so, with repeated practice, performance improves.

In oral-motor and feeding therapy, behavior modification techniques and cues are helpful in decreasing the stuffing of food and tactile defensiveness. Stuffing behavior may be caused by the child's poor sensory awareness of food in his mouth. As a behavior modification approach would not treat his sensory need, this approach should be paired with a sensory awareness program. Stuffing behavior may also be a habituated behavior, so, even though sensory awareness may improve, stuffing continues. In such a case, a behavior modification program can provide the child with a cue to attend to the amount of food in his mouth by taking one bite at a time. Initially, the therapist may use a physical cue with hand-over-hand guidance, gradually moving to an auditory or visual cue. Consistent reinforcement is given throughout this process.

When using a behavior modification program to target tactile defensiveness, consider using time segments and turntaking as strategies. A tactile stimulation program should begin in the areas best tolerated by the child, usually in the limbs. The child is often more sensitive as you approach the face and mouth. Firm, deep pressure should be used. Once oral contact is established, gradually increase the time duration of the stimulation. When stimulating the tongue with a toothbrush or tapping the cheeks, establish an interval of time by counting aloud, beginning at the easiest tolerated level. Take turns with the child so that he is able to give himself input. The child may be able to tolerate self-input easier than therapist-input.

Sensory Environment

The sensory features of the therapy environment will also impact on the fragile X child's oral-motor and feeding skills. Input is received through seven senses: auditory, visual, tactile, gustatory (taste), olfactory (smell), proprioceptive, and vestibular. For a complete review of these senses see Chapters 4 and 6. In this section, the focus is on the tactile, gustatory, olfactory, and proprioceptive senses and their relationship to oral-motor and feeding therapy. Goals include normalizing the response to sensory input, targeting hyposensitivity (lack of sensory feedback), and targeting hypersensitivity (extreme sensitivity to input). When developing therapy, consider providing a variety of sensory opportunities using foods, utensils, and equipment. Children with fragile X are often described by their parents as picky eaters. The youngsters may be unwilling to eat certain foods because of unfamiliar texture or smell.

Opportunities to experience new foods may be provided during snack time. A group snack activity may encourage the child to sample a new food a peer is eating. Foods can be selected to meet specific goals and provide the opportunity for all children in the group to taste different foods.

Foods With Sensory Variations and Textures

Foods that can be prepared and served in a variety of sensory combinations are excellent for snacks. Such flexible foods allow for making gradual changes for children who resist eating new foods. Food groups should be chosen with both mild and strong flavors and smells. Vegetables with a mild flavor, such as cucumber, can be sampled, as well as those with stronger flavors, such as broccoli. Other snacks include sweet and tart fruits (i.e., melons and grapefruit), different flavors of gum, and drinks such as apple juice.

Foods that have a variety of textures should be selected for snack time. Snacks can include: mushy or creamy foods (mashed banana, pudding); lumpy foods (cottage cheese, rice); firm, chewy foods (slim jims, firmed meats, cooked chopped vegetables); crisp or crunchy foods (potato chips, bagel chips); and sticky foods (peanut butter, marshmallows). Foods that require extended chewing, such as firm and crunchy foods, are often resisted by these children. Chewing provides proprioceptive input to the jaw that may serve to increase muscle tone and arouse sensations.

Foods consisting of more than one texture are very challenging to children with sensory deficits. Creamy and crunchy combinations, such as raw vegetables with dip or celery with peanut butter, are excellent and nutritious snacks. Foods that combine a liquid with a solid or those that produce extra juice when chewed require the child to swallow the liquid while chewing. Examples of these foods include: cereal and milk, vegetable soup, and orange slices. The child may refuse to use utensils, because the spoon or fork adds an additional texture. Experiment with spoons of various sizes and shapes with an easily tolerated food. Other snack combinations include: jello with fruit, milk shake with granola, and fruit salad.

Equipment

The equipment used in oral sensory motor therapy is chosen to provide a variety of sensory experiences during physical handling and stimulation. Many of these tools are selected to provide calming input. For example, to provide different textile sensations to the body and face, we use powder, cream, a soft terrycloth, and brushes.

Each of these is used carefully, observing the child's response and following the guidelines previously discussed in this section (i.e., type of touch, distal to proximal placement). A toothbrush and Q-tips are used to provide tactile input inside the mouth. An electric toothbrush may be used if the child can tolerate it. This input serves to increase sensory awareness.

TREATMENT FOR IMPROVED INTELLIGIBILITY

Poor speech intelligibility in boys with fragile X may be a function of phonological errors; dyspraxia; disturbed prosody including stress, intonation, rate, and juncture; or an unusual voice quality characterized by hoarseness, harshness, or inappropriate volume. This section focuses on intervention strategies to improve intelligibility. Strategies have been chosen that incorporate skill strengths in children with fragile X. These children respond well to visually presented information. The use of visual cues paired with auditory input will often increase the targeted behavior. Imitation is also a strength in children with fragile X and can be an excellent tool in teaching intelligibility. Poor intelligibility may also be a function of the sensory system seen in boys with fragile X. When their sensory system is overloaded, speech rate may increase and problems with prosody and dyspraxia may result. Techniques to help calm and organize the child's sensory system are discussed in this section.

Goals for therapy include (Novakovich, 1989, p. 30):

- Improve motor planning for speech;
- Improve production of phonetically/motorically complex words;
- Demonstrate appropriate use of suprasegmentals: rate, pitch, stress, loudness, pauses, and rhythm;
- Produce target sound in isolation, syllables, words, phrases, sentences.

Dyspraxia

The speech of boys with fragile X has been described as dyspraxic and is characterized by difficulty ordering and sequencing sounds (Chapter 5). These children have more difficulty producing sounds in connected speech than in single words. They also exhibit difficulty producing multisyllabic words. The Signed Targeted Phoneme procedure (Shelton & Garves, 1985) was developed for use with children demonstrating characteristics of developmental apraxia. It uses hand shapes from the American Manual Alphabet to visually cue the targeted sound. The visual cues are paired with a verbal model. The Adapted Cueing Technique (Klick, 1985) also uses a visual cue with an emphasis on sequential articulatory movements and the manner of speech sound production. In addition to cueing the verbal model with a sign, this program employs movement to represent manner of production and the sequence of speech sounds. These techniques may be useful in visually cueing the child to sequence sounds in multisyllabic words or in structured phrases or sentences.

The use of music and movement can also be useful tools in increasing intelligibility in fragile X boys. Choose songs with a simple rhythm, then pair gross motor movements and a series of speech sounds. These sound combinations should be meaningful, using either targeted multisyllabic words or short phrases or sentences. The Melodic Intonation Treatment program (Sparks & Holland, 1976) can be adapted for use with the fragile X child. This program was developed to improve verbal communication skills in adult aphasics and has been shown to facilitate articulation (Zoller, 1991). It uses a limited range of notes and is based on various speech prosody patterns. It is slower and more lyrical than speech. The child is required to imitate patterns accompanied by assisted hand-tapping. The slower, lyrical utterance appears to help the fragile X child focus and improve attention to auditory input. The assisted hand-tapping incorporates movement synchronized with the speech and further reinforces the rate and intonation patterns. Other gross motor movements can be paired with pitch changes and rate to target these goals.

Prosody

The spontaneous speech samples of boys with fragile X are often characterized by increased rate and unusual intonation patterns causing reduced intelligibility. In our experience, speech rate, juncture, and intonation are greatly improved when the child is calm. Slow, rhythmic, and deep input provided through the tactile, proprioceptive, and vestibular senses helps to slow down the body and calm the child (Chapter 6). Speech rate often decreases, spacing between words becomes more appropriate, and fluency improves. There is also a decrease in sound and word repetitions. Inhibitory techniques are developed in consultation with the team OT for use in the speech therapy room.

The speech therapy session usually begins with calming activities. Based on the child's sensory need that particular day and his response to the input, calming activities may be used intermittently or continuously throughout the session. Speech activities that focus on production of multisyllabic words, coarticulation of a targeted sound, or grammatical structure (past tense or plural markers) in a phrase or sentence should be paired with the calming activity. For example, work on production of the final /t/ to mark regular past tense (jumped, brushed, walked), can be done during a sensory-motor exercise. Tactile input may be given using lotion, powder, a vibrator, brushes, or other mediums. Input should be slow, rhythmical, and deep and can be applied to the arms, legs, and back. The child's response and his ability to tolerate touch must be monitored by the therapist. Observation of, or training by an occupational therapist with a sensory integration background is recommended. Calming techniques employing tactile input are discussed in greater detail in Chapter 6.

Proprioceptive input can also have a calming and organizing effect on the child's system. Techniques that may be used in the therapy room include: chair, wall, and hand-to-hand push ups; pushing or pulling heavy objects; joint compression; pressing firmly on the cheeks, forehead, chin, shoulders, and head; and biting the handle of a toothbrush. Vestibular input that is slow, steady, and rhythmic can be calming and organizing for a child. Slow and steady rocking on a rocking chair is an excellent example of a calming technique that can be done in a therapy room. Most calming techniques that use the vestibular system require suspended equipment used in an occupational therapy room. These techniques are discussed in the Occupational Therapy chapter. The vestibular system is very sensitive to overstimulation and calming techniques employing this system must be used cautiously and in consultation with an OT.

An 8-year-old fragile X boy received 30 minutes each of individual occupational therapy, speech and language therapy, and combined therapy with the occupational therapist and speech therapist. He presented with a rapid speech rate, phonological errors predominantly in connected discourse, and decreased volume. Various tactile, proprioceptive, and vestibular techniques were used with the child to help calm his system. While experimenting with various tactile mediums and body locations, the team OT discovered that the child responded best to firm brushing on the soles of his feet. This tactile and proprioceptive input served to decrease his speech rate and improve intelligibility. He learned to request feet brushing immediately on entering the therapy room. He realized that in addition to improving his intelligibility, this input also helped him to focus and attend to information (Figure 7-8). The use

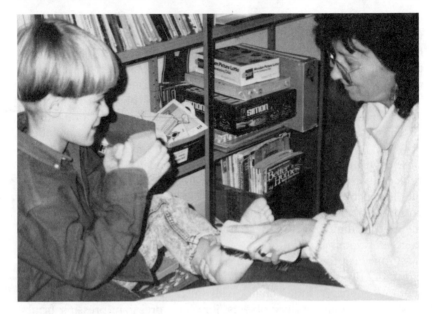

Figure 7-8. Brushing feet for calming input. Note attention and eye contact.

of calming techniques are also discussed in the auditory processing section.

Vocal Intensity

The speech volume of children with fragile X can vary by a speaker and between speakers (Newell, Sanborn, & Hagerman, 1983). In our experience, the decreased loudness of children with fragile X often interferes with intelligibility. We have also observed children who demonstrate variable loudness. One boy would initiate an utterance in a loud, intelligible voice that would quickly change and become soft, almost inaudible, and mumbling.

Poor speech volume may be related to decreased muscle tone causing insufficient breath support for phonation. Sensory integration and neurodevelopmental treatment (NDT) techniques can be used to facilitate full extension of the upper body thereby extending the rib cage and allowing increased lung capacity. Activities that encourage trunk extension include: reaching up, overhead ball throwing, or pushing up on an object. Vocalizing during the activity should be encouraged and may be rote language, such as counting or interactive language. The child with fragile X may also have difficulty motor planning the amount of air to breathe in for prolonged and smooth phonation. Proprioceptive input such as bouncing on an inner tube or jumping appears to send information to the brain about the contraction and relaxation of the diaphragm.

AUDITORY PROCESSING, EXPRESSIVE LANGUAGE, AND CRITICAL THINKING SKILLS

Boys with fragile X demonstrate language dysfunction ranging from moderate to severe receptive and expressive language delays (Newell et al., 1983). Receptive deficits may be observed as poor auditory attention, memory, and in semantic and syntactic comprehension. Behavioral characteristics such as hyperactivity and impulsivity can interfere with attention (Scharfenaker, 1990). Expressive characteristics may include excessive verbalizations, poor sequencing and organization, perseveration on word and phrases, and echolalia. This section focuses on techniques to modify the learning environment to improve receptive and expressive language and problem-solving skills. The specific learning style and the sensory system of the fragile X child needs to be considered when developing effective strategies.

Goals for comprehension of targeted information include (Novakovich, 1989, pp. 32-33):

- Demonstrate increased attention span for speech/language;
- Demonstrate comprehension of words, phrases, sentences, paragraphs, stories;
- Demonstrate comprehension of conversation;
- Follow routine directions;
- Follow novel directions;
- Demonstrate comprehension of questions: yes/no, what, who, where, whose, when, which, why, and how.

Goals for language organization include (Novakovich, 1989, pp. 36-37):

- Relate events (personal, experiential, pictured, ongoing, immediate, past, future) using: precise vocabulary, appropriate amount of detail, logical sequence of events;
- Reduce occurrence of mazing by decreasing false starts, time buyers, topic switches, circumlocutions, and excessive repetitions;
- Inhibit inappropriate verbalizations.

Goals to improve critical thinking skills include (Novakovich, 1989, pp. 39-40):

• Demonstrate comprehension and expression of categories;
• Demonstrate comprehension and expression of likenesses and differences;
• Demonstrate comprehension and expression of synonyms, opposites, associations, analogies, inferences, cause/effect relationships, and figurative language.

Learning Environment

Boys with fragile X appear disorganized and have negative reactions to changes in their environment. They become anxious and their language skills decrease during transitions and when unpredictable events occur. They may demonstrate more difficulty processing information and in their verbal expression. A structured environment in which the child knows what to expect and what is expected of him is extremely important. A calendar of daily activities can be used to organize the sequence of the day within the classroom. Photographs of team therapists and a schedule of services can be posted to alert the child for therapy. Individual schedule books may be used with older children to teach organizational skills.

While learning organizational skills is extremely important for the fragile X child, the ability to handle unpredictable events is also important for functioning within and outside the school setting. Techniques for practicing flexibility and dealing with changes include preparing the child for a change in his schedule by verbalizing, "We're going to do something different now. That's OK," or by programming unpredictable events into a schedule. Braden (1989) suggests that initially an unexpected event be inserted into the child's regular schedule at the same time each day. Such an event may include learning a new task, working with a new person, or working in an unfamiliar location. As the child becomes more comfortable with changes, the time of day variations occur can be modified. In this way, the child will not become schedule-dependent.

A behavior management program can help the child define expectations. The predictability of this program provides organization for the fragile X child. A behavior program involves the use of both positive and negative consequences for specific behaviors targeted for change, allowing the therapist to identify, monitor, and alter a specific behavior. The therapist must first identify the targeted behavior and determine the importance, severity, and frequency of the behavior. An appropriate reward for the child for production of the targeted behavior must be determined. This may be tangible, such as stickers, or verbal. If verbal reinforcement is used, however, it should be delivered in a calm and low-keyed manner to not excite or overload the child's sensory system. Initially, reinforcement should be frequent and regular, with a gradual change to intermittent reinforcement.

In the previous section, a behavior management program was mentioned as a means to decrease stuffing foods when eating. A behavior program may be used to increase attention. For example, a child can be consistently reinforced for answering a question the first time it is asked. Questions should be targeted that are within the child's skill repertoire.

Auditory and Visual Input

Children with fragile X are often hypersensitive to their environment and have difficulty screening out auditory and visual distractions. Sensory input may be distracting and can impact on the child's ability to attend to and process information and may impair verbal output. Behaviors resulting from an overload can include agitation, hyperactivity, and impulsivity.

When planning therapy activities for children with fragile X, consider the auditory distractions that may be part of the learning environment. Therapy sessions should be in an area with minimal noise. The child should not be seated near windows or high traffic areas. Fragile X children can also become overloaded by their own verbalizations. When this happens, calming techniques without verbal interaction may be helpful. Any therapist interaction and reinforcement should be soft and low-keyed. Auditory information can also be presented in a slower fashion, with pauses between phrases and sentences, particularly when giving directions.

Auditory input may be used as a tool to teach the child with fragile X. Music can be included in a child's program as a means of creating an auditory environment more conducive to learning. In an informal study, Morris (1985b) observed that using music with a regular rhythm and tempo of 60 beats per minute produced positive effects during treatment. Children became calmer and less distractable. Music set at a low volume can also be used to mask continuous distractions. Music can also be used to highlight new concepts and vocabulary (Zoller, 1991).

Visual distractions should also be monitored when planning therapy. Lighting should be of medium intensity, with no flickering or blinking lights. Posters, pictures, and other visual materials on the walls or therapy table should be limited. A carrel can be used to partition a small work area for the child. The therapist may want to sit beside or behind the child instead of across from him. The therapist can reduce the visual stimuli by cutting worksheets or by placing white paper over extraneous pictures. Color may be used to highlight important information. In a study by Zentall and Kruczek (1988), children with attention problems demonstrated improved performance when color emphasis was used to focus the child on specific information.

Cues and Prompts

Prompts are a vital part of teaching a new skill to fragile X youngsters. A prompt is the event that helps initiate a response. Types of prompts include: verbal cues, visual cues, gestural cues, motor cues, modeling, and physical assistance. Prompts can be combined. When the child begins to demonstrate improvement in his performance of the targeted skill, gradually fade the use of the prompt or change to a less structured prompt (Glendenning, 1983).

The types of cues that will be most successful are usually determined by the targeted skill and the individual's learning style. Children with fragile X appear to respond best to visual, gestural, and motor cues. Pairing a visual and motor cue with the verbal model may result in improved comprehension and expression. For example, when teaching the sequence to a story, the therapist and child can reenact the story, motorically acting out the pictures and simultaneously pairing the verbal response. Sequence stories that incorporate gross motor movement appear to elicit greater comprehension and expressive organization. Signed cues can be used to teach new concepts or vocabulary words, grammatic forms, and as reinforcement for directions. Such signals can be used to help the child expressively organize a sentence or retrieve a specific word.

Simultaneous Learning Style

Boys with fragile X tend toward a simultaneous learning style. Their academic performance is affected by the way stimuli are presented. Information processed as a gestalt rather than in parts or sequentially appears to enhance performance. When implementing therapy, consider presenting the information as a whole. For example, in a listening comprehension activity such as a story, read the whole story before asking questions. The fragile X child may be anxious to hear the conclusion and will have difficulty processing the questions that interrupt the story's flow. In experience activities (cooking, art, science experiments), first demonstrate the entire process so the child may observe the finished product or result before requiring the child to repeat portions of the experience or asking specific questions. The child with fragile X needs to know an outcome to reduce the anxiety that so often affects their performance. A simultaneous presentation allows the therapist to diminish the effects of anxiety on performance.

Curriculum, High-Interest Information, and Humor

Information that is of high interest or humorous to the child can often promote and foster learning; increase language attention, comprehension, and memory; and impact on the expressive skills of the fragile X child. Observation at school and in the home will often yield information concerning interest areas. These may range from insects and animals to fast foods or television. Therapist creativity will be needed to incorporate interests into specific goals. For example, one fragile X child was fascinated by insects. Auditory attention and comprehension goals were targeted by reading stories and creating riddles concerning insects. Nature walks and simple experiments provided activities for expressive organization and social interaction.

Classroom curriculum areas of science and social studies can be used as vehicles to teach targeted goals and provide high-interest information. Social studies units can increase the child's knowledge of the community, culture, and the geography of the world. Language therapy may focus on specific vocabulary related to an academic unit, and enhance attention and comprehension of more complex information that is, hopefully, of high interest. For example, a targeted unit was on world communities featuring Japan, Mexico, and Ghana. The classroom teacher focused on the people, location, and culture of each community. The language therapist used related materials to provide listening attention and comprehension activities. The children role-played greetings and interactions specific to each culture, with expressive language and social goals targeted.

Science units allow the child to interact with a variety of materials in their environment. Units on matter, energy, and ecology can focus on vocabulary and concept development, with experimentation allowing the child to observe a sequence of steps in proving a hypothesis. Science experiments are excellent tools for language goals such as following directions, listening attention and comprehension, expressive organization, and problem-solving.

Humor can be used as a teaching strategy with fragile X children in numerous ways. We have used humorous expressions, jokes, and comedy routines seen on television. In one case, a 10-year-old boy with fragile X could perform many of the Three Stooges' comedy routines. In therapy, we used these routines to gain attention and for reinforcement.

Sensory System

The fragile X child's ability to process and use language appears to be strongly influenced by the state of his sensory system at a given time. These children are easily overaroused and are hypersensitive to stimuli in their environment. The therapist must be aware of the fragile X child's tendency to be hyperactive and become distracted by internal and external stimuli, despite the therapist's attempt to control these factors. Optimally, the child should be calm and focused at the start of the therapy session. Since this is often unlikely with fragile X boys, calming techniques can be employed to decrease the activity level. Attention, comprehension, and expressive language are improved when the child is calm. Sensory input that is calming and organizing should be incorporated into language therapy before and during an activity (Chapters 6 and 8).

SOCIAL LANGUAGE THERAPY

Pragmatic language competence is the ability to comprehend and use verbal and nonverbal behaviors for communication. For individuals to be proficient communicators, they must be able to initiate, maintain, and terminate a conversation. They must demonstrate joint focus of attention during the interaction. Conversation serves a variety of functions. Conversational acts may be assertive or responsive and may include requests for attention, information, action, clarification, and disagreement (Fey, 1986). Social language proficiency is also dependent on the ability to comprehend and use nonverbal cues such as eye contact, gestures, facial expressions, and proximity.

Boys with fragile X demonstrate deficiencies in their pragmatic language skills. Although they are often very interested in communicating, they demonstrate difficulty with topic initiation and maintenance (Madison, George, & Moeschler, 1986; Sudhalter, Cohen, Silverman, & Wolf-Schein, 1990). Conversational speech is characterized by tangential comments, perseveration on earlier topics, and automatic phrases. Reduced eye contact is seen in most boys with fragile X (Hagerman, 1988). This section focuses on intervention strategies to improve social language skills.

Goals for therapy include (Novakovich, 1989, pp. 34-36):

- Demonstrate understanding of adult/child focus of attention;
- Gain attention in a way appropriate to the situation;
- Demonstrate comprehension and use of eye contact/facial orientation as a nonverbal social convention;
- Demonstrate comprehension and use of: distance, facial expression, gesture, and posture as nonverbal conventions;
- Demonstrate beginning knowledge of conversational skills by inhibiting vocalization when adult vocalizes;
- Initiate, maintain, and terminate a conversation;
- Use language/gestures to engage in social routines;
- Use language/gesture to engage in interactive play;
- Make direct and indirect requests for: action, information, clarification, permission, acknowledgment.

Natural Environment

Language therapy focusing on interaction in conversation and play should occur in a meaningful and experiential environment. Fey (1986) states that children should be expected to produce a targeted behavior only under conditions where there is a need to communicate. For children with fragile X, learning and practicing targeted goals in this manner allows the child to produce the behavior in a meaningful context and reduce the need for generalizations they find very difficult.

A natural environment should be chosen to facilitate the production of targeted conversational acts and enforce the use of conversational rules. Play activities should occur in a natural environment within the classroom, therapy room, or playground. The environment must be appropriate for the child's developmental level of play and interaction (Norris & Hoffman, 1990). The SLP must observe the child in order to determine his level of play and create a situation that the child understands (Westby, 1990). The therapist can encourage social language behaviors within this context. For example, a 3-year-old fragile X male was playing with a toy house, then switched toys. In an attempt to focus on topic maintenance, the SLP manipulated the house (rang doorbell, opened door) and verbalized these acts to maintain the child's interest and interaction with the toy. The SLP can also encourage the production of conversational acts during play by her willingness to interpret the child's utterance as a request and respond accordingly (Fey, 1986). For example, a 10-year-old boy with fragile X often perseverated on statements about his father's car. The SLP interpreted his comments as a means to initiate conversation.

Social language skills may also be targeted in functional activities. Natural settings outside of the classroom include a kitchen or model apartment, school offices, and places in the community such as a store, restaurant, post office, etc. Activities are developed to target conversational acts and rules. The child can initiate a conversation to request information or action: for example, in a grocery store to find an item, or in a restaurant to request a meal. In a kitchen, the child can problem-solve the steps to cook and serve breakfast including: locating objects to set the table, locating appropriate kitchen appliances and utensils for food preparation, locating food, and food preparation. Verbal and nonverbal interaction is required to complete these activities.

Whole Language

Whole language theory provides a framework for social language intervention that may be appropriate for children with fragile X. In classrooms that use a whole language approach to teaching, there is an emphasis on natural language use. The curriculum is child-centered. Activities are geared to the child's functioning level and proceed from his areas of strength. Westby (1990) states, "successful whole language programs use information about students' interests, abilities, and needs to increase oral pragmatic, semantic, syntactic, and phonemic knowledge" (p. 229). The SLP working with fragile X children should take advantage of these aspects of the whole language classroom to provide opportunities for comprehension and language use, as well as the practice of interactive language skills in a natural setting.

Modeling and Expansion

Modeling is the demonstration of a skill. Because children with fragile X demonstrate strong imitative skills, modeling can be an effective strategy. For modeling to be successful, the child must be able to observe the behavior frequently in a natural and meaningful environment. The complexity of the modeled utterance should be reduced to the child's level of understanding. While modeling has been included in this chapter as a strategy for social language, it may also be used when working on rate, prosody, and expressive language organization skills. Modeling does pose one disadvantage in pragmatic therapy in that it is a therapist-oriented strategy (Fey, 1986). Meaningfulness for the child may be decreased, because the therapist must determine the behavior to be modeled.

Expansion is a child-centered strategy, with the therapist verbally responding by repeating a child-initiated utterance and adding a few new words. The additional information may be grammatical or may provide new semantic content. Expansions can be used when the child with fragile X perseverates on a phrase or topic. Perseveration may occur when the child wants to continue a topic, but is either unsure or unable to retrieve additional information. Therapist expansion provides the child with new information to help him maintain a topic more appropriately. The therapist may need to use verbal and nonverbal prompts to help the child communicate the expanded message. Continuing with the example of the 10-year-old fragile X child, the SLP has already interpreted his perseverative comments as an initiation of conversation. Now using expansion, she helps him continue the conversation by providing related information about cars, in general. The prompts may include questions, signed cues, and pictures.

Role Playing

Piaget (1965) wrote that children use play as a natural form of expression and that role play occurs frequently in natural play. The use of role playing as a strategy in social language therapy for the fragile X child has the advantage of providing practice of a previously modeled social behavior in a natural play context. Role playing facilitates the use of interactive language behaviors, such as social routines (greetings, introductions); requests for action, information, and attention; and expression of feelings. Other language behaviors that are practiced in role playing activities include initiating, maintaining, and terminating interaction, plus turntaking skills. It is important to provide the fragile X child with opportunities to role play these behaviors with a variety of partners and in various settings. Initial activities should occur in a familiar environment with a familiar and nonthreatening partner. With a child who can read, scripts may be used as a means to rehearse these new behaviors. Role playing may focus either on the language required for interacting with peers in the classroom or with individuals in and outside the school setting. For example, activities can target the language needed to share toys, relate a message to the school secretary, or order food in a restaurant.

Eye Contact

Eye contact and body orientation are behaviors that are often deviant in males with fragile X. Poor eye contact may be related to social gaze avoidance (Cohen, Vietze, Sudhalter, Jenkins, & Brown, 1991). Fragile X boys are sensitive to gaze initiated by others. They often turn their body away from the speaker to avoid the line of gaze.

With this in mind, seating placement in small group therapy for the fragile X child should not be face to face. Seating alternatives include sitting side to side, around one side of a table, at an angle, or behind the child. Focusing on the material eliminates some of the demand for eye contact in a natural way and may reduce the sensory overload that eye contact may produce. While eye contact is difficult for many individuals with fragile X, it can be included in therapy as an isolated skill and required in activities that address other speech language goals. In a study by Kelley and Ninan (1990), an individual's satisfaction with a conversational partner's ability was observed. It was found that behaviors such as eye contact, facial attentiveness, and body orientation had more impact on satisfaction than verbal behaviors. These nonverbal and verbal social language goals can be addressed using sensory techniques for calming the child's system. For example, in targeting comprehension of facial expressions and gestures, the therapist sits across from the child and simultaneously gives deep proprioceptive input to the muscles and joints of the arms or legs. This input calms and focuses the fragile X child to facilitate eye contact and facial and body orientation.

Games can be used to establish and work on eye contact. Winking and blinking games orient the attention and gaze to the eyes without requiring interaction. Therapy activities may include counting winks or blinks or watching for which eye blinks—left or right. In a group activity, one child is chosen as the winker and the other children must look at participant's eyes to see which will wink. Determining eye color requires momentary eye contact and can be used with both familiar and less familiar individuals.

Mainstreaming

The Education for All Handicapped Children Act of 1975 (P.L. 94-142), states that handicapped children must receive an education in the "least restrictive environment." This means that students with special needs, who have been traditionally placed in self-contained classrooms or schools, are to spend as much time as possible in regular classrooms, with support from special education staff as needed. Children with fragile X benefit from integrating with students in typical classrooms, because fragile X children demonstrate strong social imitative skills (Scharfenaker, Hickman, & Braden, 1991). To focus on social skill development, mainstreaming for nonacademic periods should be encouraged. Age-appropriate peers provide the model for verbal and nonverbal social behaviors. Goldstein (1981) states that modeling is most effective when the child views the model as highly skilled and the model is the same age and sex as the child (in Fiedler & Chiang, 1989). As the child begins to imitate and use socially appropriate behaviors, the nonhandicapped peer provides natural reinforcement by maintaining the interaction. This reinforcement is more likely to occur in a mainstreamed setting than a self-contained program.

A buddy system can be used, with a nonhandicapped peer paired with the fragile X child to model socially appropriate behaviors. The buddy supports the child in both mainstreamed and self-contained settings and can also function as a peer tutor for academic activities. A higher functioning fragile X child may be mainstreamed for academic periods. Madden and Slavin (1983) report that heterogeneous placement can enhance the handicapped student's achievement when the regular class is structured to meet the needs of the child.

REFERENCES

Bangs, T.E. (1975). *Vocabulary comprehension scale.* Austin, TX: Learning Concepts.

Blank, M., Rose, S.A., & Berlin, L.J. (1978). *Preschool language assessment instrument.* Orlando: Grune and Straton.

Bobath, B. (1987, Summer). *The concept of neurodevelopmental treatment.* Neurodevelopmental treatment course, Rockville, MD (handout).

Bracken, B.A. (1984). *Bracken basic concept scale.* Columbus: Bell and Howell Company.

Braden, M. (1989, April). *Strategies for the fragile X patient.* International fragile X Conference, Denver, CO (handout).

Brownell, R. (1987). *Receptive one-word picture vocabulary test: Upper extension.* Novato, CA: Academic Therapy Publications.

Carrow-Woolfolk, E. (1985). *Test for auditory comprehension of language* (rev. ed.). Allen, TX: DLM Teaching Resources.

Cohen, I., Vietze, P., Sudhalter, V., Jenkins, E., & Brown, T. (1991). Effects of age and communication level on eye contact in fragile X males and non-fragile X autistic males. *American Journal of Medical Genetics, 38,* 498-502.

DiSimoni, F. (1978). *The token test for children.* Boston: Teaching Resources Corp.

Dunn, L.M., & Dunn, L.M. (1981). *Peabody picture vocabulary test* (rev. ed.). Circle Pines, MN: American Guidance Service.

Fey, M. (1986). *Language intervention with young children.* Boston: College-Hill Press.

Fiedler, C., & Chiang, B. (1989). Teaching social skills to students with learning disabilities. *LD Forum, 15,* 19-21.

Foster, R., Giddan, J.J., & Stark, J. (1973). *Assessment of children's language comprehension.* Palo Alto, CA: Consulting Psychologists Press.

Gardner, M.F. (1979). *Expressive one-word picture vocabulary test.* Novato, CA: Academic Therapy Publications.

Gardner, M.F. (1983). *Expressive one-word picture vocabulary test: Upper extension.* Novato, CA: Academic Therapy Publications.

Gardner, M.F. (1985). *Receptive one-word picture vocabulary test.* Novato, CA: Academic Therapy Publications.

Glendenning, N. (1983). Comparison of prompt sequences. *American Journal of Mental Deficiency, 88,* 321-325.

Goldstein, A.P. (1981). Social skills training. In A.P. Goldstein, E.G. Carr, W.S. Davidson II, & P. Weber (Eds.), *In response to aggression: Methods of control and prosocial alternatives* (pp. 159-218). New York: Pergamon Press.

Hagerman, R. (1988). Fragile X syndrome. *Early Childhood Update, 4,* 5-6.

Hammill, D.D. (1985). *Detroit tests of learning aptitude.* Austin: PRO-ED.

Hedrick, D.L., Prather, E.M., & Tobin, A.R. (1984). *Sequenced inventory of communication development.* Seattle: University of Washington Press.

Kelley, D., & Ninan, M. (1990, February). Communication skills affecting listening satisfaction. Paper presented at the Annual Meeting of the Western Speech Communication Association, Sacramento, CA.

Kirk, S.A., & Kirk, W.D. (1968). *Illinois test of psycholinguistic abilities* (rev. ed.). Champaigne: University of Illinois.

Klick, S. (1985). Adapted cuing techniques for use in treatment of dyspraxia. *Language, Speech, and Hearing Services in Schools, 16,* 256-259.

Madden, N., & Slavin, R. (1983). Mainstreaming students with mild handicaps: Academic and social outcomes. *Review of Educational Research 53,* 519-569.

Madison, L., George, C., & Moeschler, J.B. (1986). Cognitive functioning in the fragile X syndrome: A study of intellectual, memory, and communication skills. *Journal of Mental Deficiency Research, 30,* 129-148.

Morris, S.E. (1977). *Program guidelines for children with feeding problems.* Edison, NJ: Childcraft Education Corporation.

Morris, S.E. (1985a). Developmental implications for the management of feeding problems in neurologically impaired. *Seminars in Speech and Language, 6,* 293-315.

Morris, S.E. (1985b, December). Music and hemi-sync in the treatment of children with developmental disabilities. *Breakthrough,* 1-4.

Morris, S.E. (1987). Therapy for the child with cerebral palsy: Interacting frameworks. *Seminars in Speech and Language, 8,* 71-86.

Newcomer, P.L., & Hammill, D.D. (1988). *Test of language development — 2: Primary.* Austin, TX: PRO-ED.

Newell, K., Sanborn, B., & Hagerman, R. (1983). Speech and language dysfunction in the fragile X syndrome. In R.J. Hagerman & P.M.

McBogg (Eds.), *The fragile X syndrome: Diagnosis, biochemistry, and interventions* (pp. 175-200). Dillon, CO: Spectra Publishing, Inc.

Norris, J.A., & Hoffman, P. (1990). Language intervention within naturalistic environment. *Language, Speech, and Hearing Services in Schools, 21,* 72-84.

Novakovich, H. (Ed.). (1989). *Databased individual school curriculum (DISC).* Rockville, MD: Ivymount School.

Piaget, J. (1965). *The language and thought of the child.* New York: World Publishing.

Scharfenaker, S.K. (1990). The fragile X syndrome. *American-Speech-Language-Hearing Association, 32,* 45-47.

Scharfenaker, S., Hickman, L., & Braden, M. (1991). An integrated approach to intervention. In R.J. Hagerman & A.C. Silverman (Eds.), *Fragile X syndrome: Diagnosis, treatment, and research* (pp. 327-372). Baltimore, MD: Johns Hopkins University Press.

Semel, E., Wiig, E., Secord, W., & Sabers, D. (1987). *Clinical evaluation of language functions* (rev. ed.). San Antonio, TX: The Psychological Corp.

Shelton, I.S., & Garves, M. (1985). Use of visual techniques in therapy for developmental apraxia of speech. *Language, Speech, and Hearing Services in Schools, 16,* 129-131.

Shulman, B.B. (1986). *Test of pragmatic skills.* Tucson, AZ: Communication Skill Builders.

Simon, C.S. (1984). *Evaluating communicative competence.* Tucson, AZ: Communication Skill Builders.

Sparks, R.W., & Holland, A.L. (1976). Method: Melodic intonation therapy for aphasia. *Journal of Speech and Hearing Disorders, 41,* 287-297.

Sudhalter, V., Cohen, I., Silverman, W., & Wolf-Schein, E. (1990). Conversational analysis of males with fragile X, Down syndrome, and autism: Comparison of the emergence of deviant language. *American Journal of Mental Retardation, 94,* 431-441.

Westby, C.E. (1990). The role of the speech-language pathologist in whole language. *Language, Speech, and Hearing Services in Schools, 21,* 228-237.

Zachman, L., Jorgensen, C. Hiusingh, R., & Barrett, M. (1984). *Test of Problem Solving.* Moline, IL: Linguisystems.

Zentall, S., & Kruczek, T. (1988). The attraction of color for active attention-problem children. *Exceptional Children, 54,* 357-362.

Zimmerman, I.L., Steiner, V.G., & Pond, R.E. (1979). *Preschool language scale* (rev. ed.). San Antonio, TX: The Psychological Corporation.

Zoller, M. (1991). Use of music activities in speech-language therapy. *Language, Speech, and Hearing Services in Schools, 22,* 272-276.

ADDITIONAL READINGS

Ayres, A.J. (1974). The development of sensory integrative therapy and practice. Dubuque: Kendall/Hunt Publishing.

Ayres, A.J., & Mailloux, Z. (1981). Influence of sensory integration procedures on language development. *The American Journal of Occupational Therapy, 35,* 383-390.

Brooks, A., & Benjamin, B. (1989). The use of structural role play therapy in the remediation of grammatical deficits in language delayed children. *Journal of Childhood Communication Disorders, 12,* 171-186.

Clark, F.A., & Steingold, L.R. (1982). A potential relationship between occupational therapy and language acquisition. *The American Journal of Occupational Therapy, 36,* 42-44.

Cowan, M.K. (1986, September). Occupational therapy in an intensive speech and language program. *Sensory Integration Special Interest Section Newsletter,* 1-2.

Ellenwood, A., & Felt, D.L. (1989). Attention-deficit/hyperactivity disorder: Management and intervention approaches for the classroom teacher. *LD Forum, 15,* 15-17.

Goodman, K.S., Smith, E.B., Meredith, R., & Goodman, Y.M. (1987). *Language and thinking in school: A whole language curriculum.* New York: Richard C. Owen Publishers, Inc.

Hacker, B., & Ballard, D. (1986, September). Verbal and developmental dyspraxia: A case study. *Sensory Integration Special Interest Section Newsletter,* 1, 3.

Hargrove, P. (1989). Modifying the prosody of a language-impaired child. *Language, Speech, and Hearing Services in Schools, 20,* 245-258.

King, D.F., & Goodman, K.S. (1990). Whole language: Cherishing learners and their language. *Language, Speech, and Hearing Services in Schools, 21,* 221-227.

Kirby, J., & Robinson, G. (1987). Simultaneous and successive processing in reading disabled children. *Journal of Learning Disabilities, 20,* 243-252.

Norris, J.A., & Damico, J.S. (1990). Whole language in theory and practice: Implications for language intervention. *Language, Speech, and Hearing Services in Schools, 21,* 212-220.

Spekman, N.J., & Roth, E.R. (1984). Intervention strategies for learning disabled children with communication disorders. *Learning Disability Quarterly, 5,* 429-437.

Westby, C.E. (1980). Assessment of cognitive and language abilities through play. *Language, Speech, and Hearing Services in Schools, 11,* 154-168.

Windeck, S.L., & Laurel, M. (1989, March). A theoretical framework combining speech-language therapy with sensory integration treatment. *Sensory Integration Special Interest Section Newsletter,* 1-5.

8

COMBINED TREATMENT

Using combined occupational therapy and speech and language therapy to address sensory, motor, speech, and language goals can help both OTs and SLPs achieve faster results with greater generalization. Aspects of the occupational therapy program are related to aspects of the speech and language program in a reciprocal way: improvement on either set of objectives impacts on the other. For example, normalizing sensation inside the mouth may be a goal of the occupational therapist that can lead to acceptance of a greater variety of foods. The reverse, however, is also true: foods of varying texture, presented as a teaching experience during the course of working on a language unit, can be selected on the basis of enhancing acceptance. Another example involves the auditory processing area: improvement in the comprehension of auditory directions (a language goal) will facilitate the child's ability to carry out motor directions in OT, and performing motor activities in OT adds meaning to such language concepts as *over, under, fast, slow,* etc.

An important aspect of combined therapy is growth and education for the therapists. Working together promotes learning from each other and provides each therapist with a broader perspective from which to consider and treat the child. For children with fragile X, this holistic approach is especially important because their areas of disability are so highly interrelated.

RATIONALE FOR COMBINED TREATMENT

Combined occupational/speech and language therapy is based on the assumption that the integrity of the sensory-motor system of the child is closely related to the development of normal speech and language skills. Research into the nature of this relationship addresses three major areas: the connection between movement and speech and language, the effects of sensory (especially vestibular) input on speech and language, and the speculative physiological and phylogenetic relationship between the vestibular system and the auditory system. A brief review of the literature will address these three areas.

Movement and the Development of Speech and Language

Speech and language development correlates with the development of motor skills. A baby's early movements are coordinated with the melody of speech (Remling, 1990). Speech is a motor activity requiring coordination of complex movements. It requires normal muscle tone, normal movement patterns, normal timing of movement, good positioning, and coordination of respiration and phonation (Windeck & Laurel, 1989). These areas have previously been discussed as deficits in fragile X children (Chapters 4 & 5). Windeck and Laurel (1989) also propose that postural mechanisms facilitate correct sound production and that correct sound production facilitates and reinforces postural mechanisms in a sensory-motor-sensory feedback loop. Ayres (in Kelly, 1987) says that the sensation arising from movement stimulates the areas of the brain involved in making speech sounds. Children with severe articulation disorders appear to have more motor problems. This may be explained by the theory postulating that for a child with motor dysfunction, a greater percentage of energy in the central nervous system is required to maintain balance and coordination, leaving less to be devoted to the learning and production of language. The fundamental patterns of speech are built on basic body postures that lead to the development of the sequential, differentiated motor movements needed for speech sound production (Kelly, 1987). Children who have problems in some early stages of postural development (due to low muscle tone and tactile defensiveness, for example) are at risk for developing abnormal communication patterns. Children with fragile X syndrome fall into this group.

Receptively, auditory impulses are processed by auditory nuclei in the brain stem and also travel to other brain stem areas and to the cerebellum, where the input is further mixed with motor messages (Windeck & Laurel, 1989). This implies that auditory information routed to cortical processing areas is not purely auditory, but is at least partially dependent on motor information to have meaning. A child appears to perceive sound sequences in terms of his own motor patterns (Kelly, 1987). Because children with fragile X have difficulty with motor sequencing skills, their auditory processing and intelligibility may be compromised. Robinson (1977) proposed a link between activity (play) and language acquisition (in Clark & Steingold, 1982). A child first acquires concepts through action and experience, and linguistic symbols are then "mapped" onto what is already known. Piaget suggests that sensory-motor skill develops prior to language and the child's act of physical exploration stimulates the development of language concepts (in Hong & Kewley, 1989). Rider (1974) found that children with significant language problems (dysphasic children) had more abnormal reflex responses than typical children and also more than children who had only articulation problems.

Oral sensory and motor problems in children with fragile X may also be explained by the relationship of movement and speech skills. Morris (1982a, 1982b) says that the rhythmicity of oral feeding movements and that of speech production may be related (in Iammatteo, Trombly, & Loecke, 1990). Research into oral-motor problems, such as drooling, indicates that such problems have a sensory as well as a motor component (Iammatteo, et al., 1990; Weiss-Lambrou, Tetreault, & Dudley, 1989). Fragile X children, who often have difficulty with chewing and toleration of foods in the mouth (due to low tone and tactile defensiveness), have problems with rhythmical speech (Chapter 5). Hickman (1989) also mentions that stability, movement, and rhythm experienced by the body affect rhythmic speech patterns. Cowan (1986) cites poor muscle tone, postural instability, postural fatigue, and difficulty with neck control as affecting oral-motor skill and respiration for speech.

Sensory Input and Language Development

Many authors have proposed a relationship between sensory (especially vestibular-proprioceptive) input and language disorders. Remling (1990) writes that an infant's first sounds are in response to autonomic experiences (sensory input). Kelly (1987) suggests three ways in which vestibular stimulation may affect language:

1. Through direct connections between the vestibular system end-organs (the semicircular canals) and the language centers in the cerebral cortex.

2. Through increased arousal, attention, and motivation as a result of effects on the reticular activating system and/or the limbic system.
3. Through influencing hemispheric specialization which leads to more efficient language development.

The ability to use language is not just a cognitive function, but depends on central nervous system organization at all levels, from brain stem to cortex (Stilwell, Crowe, & McCallum, 1978; Windeck & Laurel, 1989). Speech and language skill acquisition has frequently been linked to vestibular dysfunction. Ayres (in Clark & Steingold, 1982) states that provision of tactile and vestibular stimulation can enhance the learning disabled child's ability to organize sensory input and plan motor output (speech), and that therapy for children with language disorders should involve not only auditory but also tactile and especially vestibular input. Ayres and Mailloux (1981) report gains in receptive and expressive language in children with sensory processing disorders after treatment with sensory integrative therapy in OT. Other authors (Ayres, 1972: Ayres & Tickle, 1980; Brashear & Berger, 1987; Kantner, Kantner, & Clark, 1982; Magrun, Ottenbacher, McCue, & Keefe, 1981; Ray, King, & Grandin, 1988; Weeks, 1979b) report similar improvements in language skills after vestibular input. Children with depressed postrotary nystagmus, an indicator of vestibular dysfunction, appear to demonstrate greater gains in language as a result of sensory integrative treatment. For children with fragile X syndrome, vestibular dysfunction is often a significant problem. Van Housen-Selley (1987) observed that the most common gross motor deficits seen in her experience with fragile X children are those requiring balance, a vestibular function. Schaff (1985) found that children with a history of otitis media demonstrated more vestibular disorders: a significant finding in view of the prevalence of otitis media in young children with fragile X. Low muscle tone, also a common problem in fragile X, is related to vestibular function and was found by Ottenbacher (1978) to be related to postrotary nystagmus (PRN). Praxis, another area of disability in fragile X, is also related to the vestibular system (Rider, 1974). Cowan (1986) found that diminished balance reactions, poor bilateral coordination and decreased PRN, all deficits seen in the fragile X population, were indicators of vestibular dysfunction. Research showed that treatment via this sensory channel resulted in improved attention, body awareness, and motor planning, all of which affect speech and language development.

Physiological Relationship Between Language and Sensory Centers

The end-organs for vestibular input are the semicircular canals located in the inner ear. They are embryologically and anatomically part of the peripheral auditory system, so it would seem logical to speculate that sensory input to one system might affect the other (Weeks, 1979a.) Kelly (1987) further explains this relationship by stating that both vestibular and auditory stimulation activate the same neural structures and that both systems respond to vibration (including sound). Auditory receptors in the brain appear to have evolved from primitive gravity receptors (Kelly 1987) and the semicircular canals, filled with fluid and covering three planes, are primary indicators of the body's relation to gravity. Sensory input does not travel to the cortex uninterrupted: the brain stem serves to integrate sensation from various systems. It has convergent neurons which require input from more than one sensory system in order to transmit impulses. At this level, for example, auditory input may be "mixed" with vestibular and proprioceptive input in order for meaningful transmission and interpretation to occur (Windeck & Laurel, 1989). More research into phylogenetic and physiologic connections between the auditory system and the vestibular system is needed, but the evidence to date suggests that such a connection exists, and provides an explanation for the treatment results cited by so many researchers and clinicians.

Implications for Combined Treatment

The research cited leads to the conclusion that combining sensory-motor and speech and language therapy is more effective than providing the two treatments in isolation. Combined treatment has been recommended for speech-language delayed and motor-impaired children in general (Campbell, McInerney, & Cooper, 1984; Clark & Steingold, 1982; Hacker & Ballard, 1986; Hong & Kewley, 1989; Kelly, 1987; Remling, 1990; Sene & Fisher, 1985; Stilwell, et al., 1978; and Windeck & Laurel, 1989), and for children with fragile X in particular (Burns & Hickman, 1989; Fisher, 1990; Gelman, 1991; Haldy, 1987; Hickman, 1989; Scharfenaker, Hickman, & Braden, 1991; and Van Housen-Selley, 1987). These authors feel that children in combined treatment make greater and faster gains, that it (1) allows children to see language in action, (2) promotes full use of gross and fine motor activities, (3) adds the component of meaning and purpose to movement, (4) contributes to professional growth and understanding of the child as a whole person, and (5) allows for more adult modeling and behavioral support. Windeck and Laurel (1989) stress the reciprocal nature of combined treatment: a child's improvements in sensory integration improve the course of his acquisition of speech and language, and his increased speech and language skills also positively affect his sensory processing and motor development. Hickman (1989, p. 15) refers to combined treatment as "pulling the body and mind together." The remainder of this chapter will focus on combined treatment models and procedures drawn from our clinical experience. Clinicians using combined treatment need to keep data and begin to do more formal research on the use of this treatment design.

FACTORS INVOLVED IN USING COMBINED TREATMENT MODELS

Combined occupational/speech/language therapy can be approached in several different ways, which are discussed in detail in the next section. There are, however, some factors to consider in using any or all of these models. We have divided these factors into **extrinsic** and **intrinsic** considerations.

Extrinsic elements such as administrative support, caseload size, availability of personnel, and physical environment enter in to decisions to use combined treatment. Ideally these factors could be arranged or changed to allow client need, alone, to dictate the use of this therapeutic model; however, these extrinsic considerations are a very real aspect of service delivery. Combined treatment requires time—often a scarce commodity for therapists. The allocation of extra time to put a combined model into practice requires administrative support. Clinicians often must present their supervisors with evidence for the rationale behind joint therapy. We hope the information in this book will be helpful. Caseload size also has an impact on flexibility of service delivery models. Although use of combined treatment may initially be difficult to establish because of large caseloads, the extra effort required in the beginning may eventually result in more efficient use of time and personnel. Some clinicians may work in areas where both OT and speech and language therapy are not available. A speech-language pathologist who serves children in a location where OT is not provided is faced with the difficult challenge of increasing the sensory motor component of her therapy without that direct support. We hope that this book will provide some direction for both OTs and speech-language pathologists who do not have many opportunities to interact. In addition, the physical set-up for therapy may be small, under-equipped, or otherwise impractical for combined treatment. However, these conditions may be overcome through tenacity and creativity if the therapists believe in the eventual benefits.

Intrinsic factors are the most important considerations in designing a service delivery model incorporating combined treatment. Client need should be primary. Many goals may be addressed through combined therapy. Clinicians must determine the following information when deciding on a model of service delivery that may include combined treatment:

1. How does sensory input affect the child's attention, organization, level of anxiety, and verbal output?
2. How do gross motor skills affect the child's experience in relation to their development of language concepts?
3. How do fine motor abilities affect the child's manual, gestural, or written communication?
4. How do oral sensory and motor issues affect the child's eating and articulation skills?

If the child appears to demonstrate significant connection between underlying sensory-motor factors and speech and language skills, some form of joint therapy should be considered. The magnitude of needs in fragile X and the holistic learning style of this population are support for a combined approach.

MODELS OF COMBINED TREATMENT

To meet the needs of every child, including and especially those with fragile X, we recommend a combined treatment model. In our experience, there is a natural continuum of types of combined treatment. Clinicians should consider all the models when choosing the most appropriate approach for an individual child or for specific goals within one child's program. The types of combined OT/SPL treatment are:

1. **Consultative:** This is probably where most therapists begin to interact: talking to each other about mutual children. Consultation often takes place informally. On a more formal level, regular staffings are often a forum for asking questions, sharing problems, or requesting reinforcement of certain goals by the other therapist. Consultation may be thought of as both the simplest and the most advanced form of combined treatment: eventually both therapists may become so familiar with each others' disciplines that

problems may be addressed through verbal consultation that may have previously required observation or actual experience.

2. **Observational:** When one therapist observes another, techniques and objectives can be demonstrated that may be difficult to convey through verbal description. Scheduling of observation time often begins as an outgrowth of consultation. While observation is time-consuming for the observing therapist, who is pulled away from providing direct treatment, the benefits of seeing rather than talking about issues may outweigh the time-crunch factor. Also, the observational model does not require prior joint planning time; it can be done on the spur of the moment when a therapist has some unexpected free time.

3. **Side-by-Side:** In this model, the OT and SLP are working together with a child or group of children, but each therapist has separate goals and equal responsibilities for different components of the activity. There is not much overlap of goals in the use of this model; rather, a common activity is used as a vehicle to address two sets of objectives. Either or both (alternating) therapists may lead the lesson.

4. **Supportive:** In the supportive model, one therapist acts as a facilitator to enable the other therapist to address her goals more effectively. One therapist usually leads the activity, with the facilitating therapist assuming a secondary role. However, if problems occur in trying to achieve a specific outcome, the supporting therapist may temporarily step in and take the lead to establish a more facilitory learning environment.

5. **Transdisciplinary:** In this model, both the OT and SLP are responsible for planning the session and establishing objectives. Both share equally in providing sensory motor and language input during the session. To be truly transdisciplinary, the two therapists should be indistinguishable to an observer.

Within each of these models there are levels and variations based on the therapists' knowledge and experience with combined treatment. It is important to know one's own limits as a transdisciplinary therapist and to recognize "red flags" (such as overstimulation) and react appropriately by seeking help.

EXAMPLES OF COMBINED TREATMENT

Examples of combined occupational/speech and language therapy are presented, based on the treatment models outlined above. It is important to remember that although consultative, observational, side-by-side, supportive, and transdisciplinary treatment may be thought of as a hierarchy in terms of their complexity, all are valid methods of co-treatment. Some objectives may be best suited to one model, some to another. Our goals are to provide a framework for OTs and SLPs to increase their comfort level with many different co-treatment options and to enhance the clinician's ability to meet the needs of fragile X and other children in their caseloads.

Consultative and Observational

Sharing respective knowledge with and learning from each other are the primary descriptors of interaction at these levels of combined treatment. Occupational and speech-language therapists who interact in these ways begin to try innovations in treatment and to be aware of the rationale for some techniques they may already use instinctively. The OT, for example, may approach the SLP with the problem that the fragile X child is having difficulty following directions in OT. The SLP may suggest techniques such as:

- Reduction of language complexity;
- Use of visual or manual (signed) cues;
- Use of shorter utterances;
- Allowing the child with fragile X to follow another child rather than go first; and
- Organizing the task holistically, not sequentially, with the end-result made clear to the child before he begins.

The speech-language therapist, in turn, may go to the OT because the child with fragile X refuses to participate in a language experience activity, such as making play-doh. The OT would be able to help by:

- Explaining tactile defensiveness;
- Recommending preparatory activities such as firm input to the hands with a brush or washcloth;
- Suggesting proprioceptive activities involving the hands;

- Providing advance explanation of the activity;
- Defining time limits for participation;
- Making the play-doh more tolerable in texture by adding flour;
- Adding color or smell components to the activity; and
- Focusing on the end product rather than on the tactile experience itself.

After sharing information and suggestions, it often becomes clear that the two therapists need to see first hand what the other is doing, setting up a natural need to observe each other. In the first example, the OT may not know how to use sign cues or how to reduce the number of critical elements in a direction. The speech therapist may be uncertain of how to use a brush on the child's hands. Table 8-1 illustrates more examples of common deficits in fragile X and how the OT and SLP can help each other deal with them at the consultative and/or observational level of co-treatment.

Side-by-Side Treatment

Functional, pragmatic, curriculum-based, and community activities often present problems for both the OT and SLP in terms of achieving the full therapeutic potential of the activity. The side-by-side treatment model is useful because it allows observation and learning to take place while both therapists are treating children. It permits both therapists to address a number of objectives and to see the other therapist doing the same. Both therapists see the child and the activity holistically and from beginning to end. For example, a science unit on simple machines may be addressed by the OT and SLP in order to carry over a classroom curriculum area into the therapeutic language and sensory motor areas. Within this unit a specific activity could be building a saw horse in order to compare the use of one pulley versus two pulleys for lifting weights. During the building activity, the SLP would address vocabulary, inferential questions and answers, and comparison statements. The OT would address the sawing, nailing and positioning. By using the side-by-side therapy model, the full spectrum of activity components are more meaningfully presented than if one therapist were leading the lesson alone. The language components add meaning and purpose to the motor components and vice versa. The children have an opportunity to participate in a complete activity—an important consideration for those with fragile X. Table 8-2 provides more examples of treatment activities using the side-by-side model.

TABLE 8-1. Examples of Co-Treatment: Consultative/Observational Model

THERAPIST INTERACTION	PROBLEM	ORIGIN	SUGGESTED STRATEGIES
SLP consults OT	Child will not stay seated	Sensory	Incorporate more movement into therapy session: • Have child go get materials periodically • Have child pick up pictures from floor instead of table • Have child march (stamp feet) while getting materials (for proprioceptive input) Give input before asking child to sit: • Wall push-ups • Chair push-ups • Heavy work (lifting, carrying, pushing, pulling) Use alternative seating: • Rocking chair • Therapy ball • Beanbag chair • Wedge
SLP consults OT	Child mouths fingers and materials	Sensory	Provide more appropriate ways to get oral input: • Chewing gum • Food with firm texture and/or strong taste • Toothbrushing • Biting more appropriate items Reduce cognitive demands of task (mouthing may be a sign of stress)
SP consults OT	Child has poor posture—leans on table, falls out of chair	Sensory	Explain low muscle tone Use alternative seating for more support: • Rifton chair (Fig. 8-1) • Chair adapted to provide built-up sides and footrest (Fig. 7-2) • Seatbelt or wrapping around waist (Fig. 8-2) • Dysem on chair seat (Fig. 8-2) Preparatory input to raise tone: • Bounce on Hippity-Hop • Bounce on therapy ball (Fig. 7-3) • Bounce on trampoline • Jump down hall to room

(continued)

TABLE 8-1.   *(continued)*

OT consults SLP	Excessive verbalization, not entirely eliminated by sensory calming techniques	Language	Explain anxiety factor Give child more information about what is going to happen: • Include picture, print, or signed cues Give child information about, or show him what the end-result of the activity will be
OT consults SLP	Child's speech is unintelligible	Language	Explain prosody and dysprosodic features of fragile X speech which have a negative impact on intelligibility (rate, fluency, loudness, rhythm) Use slower and more rhythmical speech as a model for the child Use gestures and sign language Be calm and quiet when presenting activities Give sentence completion tasks rather than direct questions Combine speech with a rhythmic motor activity

Supportive Model

Co-treatment utilizing the supportive therapy model usually takes place in a sensory motor environment. One therapist is working to accomplish an objective in her area and requires support to achieve greater success. The supporting therapist has objectives in mind also, but her goals are foundational and facilitative. By working together in the supportive model, both therapists are developing skills that will help them become more transdisciplinary and able to facilitate goals for themselves. For example, working on rate of speech with a fragile X child is a goal which lends itself well to supportive treatment. The SLP wants the child to slow down to increase intelligibility. The OT helps by providing combinations of controlled sensory input to calm the child's sensory system. The task presented by the SLP might be for the child to describe simple pictures, with the goal that all the words will be understood. The SLP provides the visual stimuli (pictures). The first facilitative task of the OT would be to decide where to position the child and the picture and to determine the equipment to be used to provide input. The OT may, for example, place the child on a platform swing and provide calming vestibular input (Figure 8-4). The OT could also provide firm tactile and proprioceptive input (Figure 8-5), and she could control the sensory environment in the room through the use

TABLE 8-2.   Examples of Co-Treatment: Side by Side Model

ACTIVITY	SPEECH AND LANGUAGE GOALS	OCCUPATIONAL THERAPY GOALS
Cooking: snacks, meals, bag lunches, special occasions	Vocabulary Concept development Sequencing Reasoning/problem-solving Pragmatic language Auditory processing: following directions Oral-motor	Bilateral integration and coordination for physical manipulation of tools and utensils Sensory defensiveness: toleration of smell, taste, and feel of foods Motor planning Balance: carry items Hand strength: mixing, cutting, kneading Activities of daily living (ADL): acquiring a useful life skill
Self-care and Grooming: washing, brushing hair, brushing teeth, dressing, selecting and caring for clothing (Fig. 8-3)	Vocabulary Concept development Oral-motor Sequencing Reasoning/problem-solving Pragmatic language	Sensory processing Fine motor skills Eye-hand coordination Motor planning Hand strength Body awareness Range of motion ADL
Community Activity: restaurant, supermarket, travel training, recreation, and leisure activities	Pragmatic language Reasoning/problem-solving Auditory processing: language comprehension Expressive language organization	ADL Sensory processing Perceptual skills: locating specific places in the community Fine motor: money, coin slots, tickets, plastic bags in supermarket

of light, color, or music. The OT can also combine inputs—for example, pulling or pushing on the ropes of the swing (proprioception) while seated or lying in prone (vestibular).

In another therapy session, the SLP might be a supporting therapist to the OT. The activity could be an obstacle course, which the OT has constructed for the child to work on motor planning. The SLP helps by providing descriptive language concepts that help the child improve praxis. Hearing the vocabulary of climbing, balancing, adds position in space add meaning to the child's movements and helps him generalize motor skills to new situations. Language provides a link in a new motor task that enables the child to better figure out how to approach it. An obstacle course without this language component is sensory motor input, but not therapy for motor planning. With the fragile X child who may not have the motor planning ability to do the obstacle course, the SLP helps set a slower pace to allow time for language organization to facilitate his

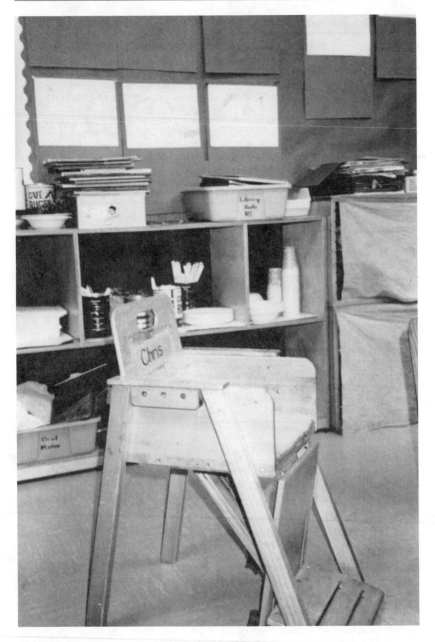

Figure 8-1.   Rifton chair.

motor performance. See Table 8-3 for more examples of the supportive model.

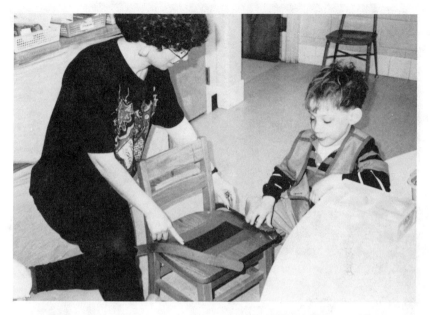

Figure 8-2.   Chair adapted with Dycem™ and seatbelt.

Transdisciplinary Model

It is difficult to give specific examples of the transdisciplinary model. All the activities previously mentioned can be transdisciplinary if the two therapists can comfortably exchange roles and equipment and/or can perform both roles when treating the child alone. Transdisciplinary treatment can be approached in two ways: through a total classroom model or in the treatment room. The total transdisciplinary classroom format requires that all staff be able to observe and learn from each other and treat children at the same time. For example, at circle time, the leader addresses language skills and other staff work on helping the children attend, respond, and maintain good body position. The next day, staff roles may be reversed. The OT and SLP (and teachers) must all be comfortable with all aspects of such activities for the transdisciplinary model to be effective. In the therapy room, either OT or speech-language, transdisciplinary treatment may be conducted by either therapist working alone, as long as she is fulfilling both roles, or by two therapists working interchangeably. Transdisciplinary treatment is not an all or nothing model: Therapists may be transdisciplinary for one goal or area or child, but not for others. It is also not necessarily always the best model for every treatment goal or every child.

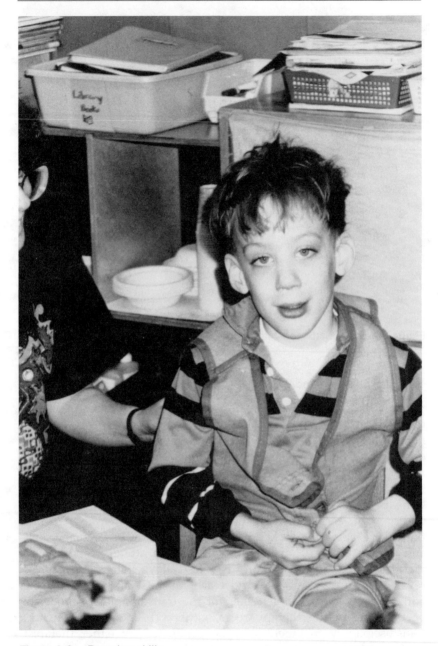

Figure 8-3.   Dressing skills.

Often, however, working toward transdisciplinary treatment is a means of growing towards treating the child holistically. With the

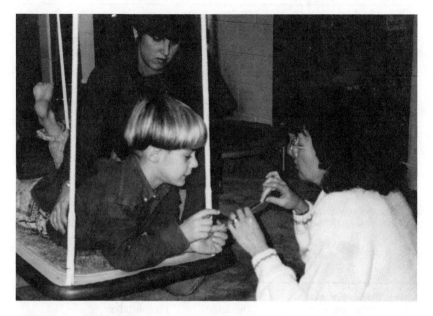

Figure 8-4. Vestibular input during language activity.

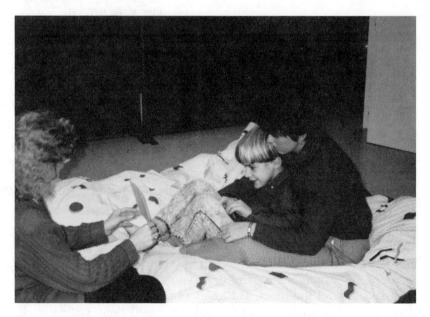

Figure 8-5. Tactile and proprioceptive input during language activity.

TABLE 8-3.   Examples of Co-Treatment: Supportive Model

ACTIVITY	PRIMARY GOALS	SUPPORTIVE GOALS AND TECHNIQUES
Child on rotary swing; SLP asks child to listen to a riddle and choose the answer from an array of Lotto cards. Child revolves or rotates to OT, directs OT to place chosen card on large Lotto board using spatial prepositions (top, middle, bottom, left, right)	Speech and Language: Auditory comprehension, expressive language	Goal (OT): Improved processing of vestibular input Techniques (OT): Platform or net swing for vestibular input
Child in cloud; SLP presents pictures and asks child to create sentences about them	Speech and Language: Decrease excessive verbalizations, increase organization of expressive language	Goal (OT): Improved focus and attention Techniques (OT): Platform or net swing for vestibular input
Making a simple breakfast, such as instant oatmeal	Occupation Therapy: Problem-solving, ADL skill building	Goal (SLP): Language organization Techniques (SLP): Visual cues via chart; chart of additional strategies for child to try (ask teacher for help, watch peers); prior verbal rehearsal
Child straddles barrel; OT facilitates reaching across midline to get food picture and place in appropriate category pile (breakfast, lunch, or dinner)	Occupational Therapy: Bilateral integration	Goal (SLP): Categorization of foods Techniques (SLP): Give purpose to body rotation activity

fragile X population, as we have said before, this is a critical concept. (Figures 8-6 and 8-7).

Example of Transdisciplinary Treatment: Two Therapists

The OT and SLP are working with a fragile X boy and another child with sensory integration dysfunction. In the OT room, a "road" has been constructed on the floor with tape lane outlines and large blocks placed to create turns. The children are positioned in prone on scooterboards and are required to negotiate along the road and around the turns. The goals of this part of the activity are trunk extension, motor planning, and increased tone. Each turn in the road goes between two blocks. On each block is a picture of an item and at each turn the children have to identify the pictures and describe their similarities and differences. In addition to this

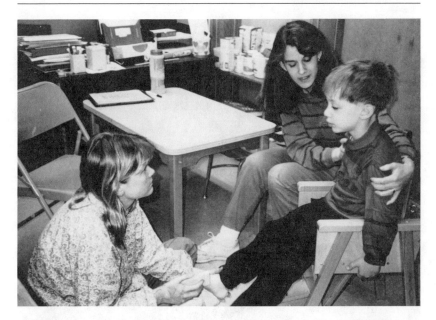

Figure 8-6. Transdisciplinary treatment. Note input to feet, shoulders, and self-directed input via chair pull-up.

language skill, the children also have to ask each other questions about the pictures. Both the OT and SLP are working on facilitation of the language and sensory-motor goals.

Example of Transdisciplinary Treatment—One Therapist

The SLP is doing language testing with a fragile X boy. He loses attention and gets up from his chair. The therapist does not respond to his behavior as a "behavior problem": instead, she recognizes his need for sensory input and immediately gives him deep pressure to his arms and hands, then gives him a dry washcloth to hold and stroke his own face and hands. He sits down and resumes the test. A speech-language therapist with less transdisciplinary orientation might not have recognized what had been truly going on in the situation and may have made it worse by placing purely behavioral demands on the child.

Transdisciplinary Treatment Examples: Guess Who?

1. Picture cards describing the sequence of the day's treatment activities are presented, using visual and auditory input to prepare the child for the session.

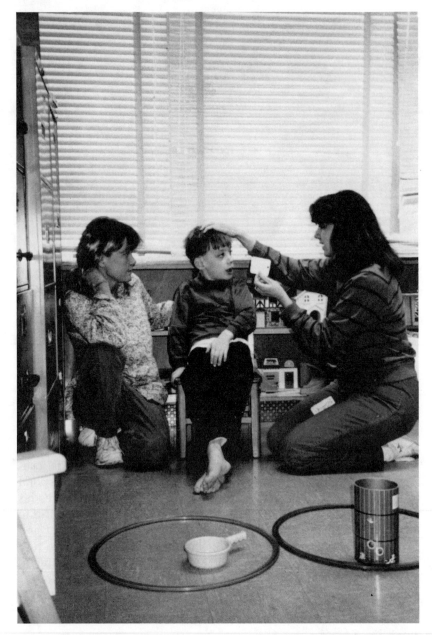

Figure 8-7. Transdisciplinary treatment. Note proprioceptive input to head.

2. A spinner game is used: the spinner lands on a preposition and the child then has to find a piece of equipment to go *on, in, under,* etc.

3. A large box of dry rice and beans contains small buried objects. Descriptive vocabulary is practiced in advance and then the child must locate an object in the box and describe it before pulling it out.

CONCLUSIONS

Combined OT/SLP treatment can be an efficient and effective therapy model for fragile X and other children who have significant and interrelated sensory, motor, and language needs. Although some research exists documenting the benefits of co-treatment, more data is needed. Many therapists are doing combined treatment and hopefully are beginning to document their methods and results. In our experience, every therapist who has tried any of the various co-treatment models has become eager to learn and do more. The more holistic we all become, the more effective will be our treatment of children, especially those with fragile X syndrome.

REFERENCES

Ayres, A.J. (1972). Improving academic scores through sensory integration. *Journal of Learning Disabilities, 5,* 23-28.

Ayres, A.J., & Mailloux, Z. (1981). Influence of sensory integration procedures on language development. *American Journal of Occupational Therapy, 35,* 383-390.

Ayres, A.J., & Tickle, L.S. (1980). Hyper-responsivity to touch and vestibular stimuli as a predictor of positive response to sensory integration procedures by autistic children. *American Journal of Occupational Therapy, 34,* 375-381.

Brashear, R.N., & Berger, P.N. (1987, March). Inter-disciplinary collaboration in a school sensory integration program. *Sensory Integration Special Interest Section Newsletter, 1,* 4.

Burns, E., & Hickman, L. (1989). Integrated therapy in a summer camping experience for children with fragile X syndrome. *Sensory Integration News, 17,* 1-3.

Campbell, P.H., McInerney, W.F., & Cooper, M.A. (1984). Therapeutic programming for students with severe handicaps. *American Journal of Occupational Therapy, 38,* 594-602.

Chu, S.K.H. (1991, September). Sensory integration and autism. *Sensory Integration Quarterly,* 3-6.

Clark, F.A., & Steingold, L.R. (1982). A potential relationship between occupational therapy and language acquisition. *American Journal of Occupational Therapy, 36,* 42-44.

Cowan, M.K. (1986, September). Occupational therapy in an intensive speech and language program. *Sensory Integration Special Interest Section Newsletter,* 1-2.

Fisher, M.A. (1990). *What is fragile X syndrome?* Fragile X Association of Michigan, 1786 Edinborough Drive, Rochester Hills, MI, 48306.

Gelman, S. (1991, Spring). An interdisciplinary approach to educating children with fragile X. *Fragile X Southeast News,* 3-4.

Hacker, B., & Ballard, D. (1986, September). Verbal and developmental dyspraxia. *Sensory Integration Special Interest Section Newsletter,* 1-3.

Haldy, M. (1987, December). A summer day camp experience for children with fragile X syndrome: A case study. *Sensory Integration Special Interest Section Newsletter,* 10.

Hickman, L. (1989). Fragile X syndrome and sensory integrative therapy. *Sensory Integration International News,* 17, 14-15.

Hong, C.S., & Kewley, C. (1989). Prelinguistic skills and occupational therapy. *British Journal of Occupational Therapy,* 52, 336-338.

Iammetteo, P.A., Trombly, C., & Luecke, L. (1990). The effect of mouth closure on drooling and speech. *American Journal of Occupational Therapy,* 44, 686-691.

Kantner, R.M., Kantner, B., & Clark, D.L. (1982). Vestibular stimulation effect on language development in mentally retarded children. *American Journal of Occupational Therapy,* 36, 36-41.

Kelly, G. (1987). Occupational therapy for speech and language disordered children: A sensory integrative approach. *British Journal of Occupational Therapy,* 50, 128-131.

Magrun, W.M., Ottenbacher, K., McCue, S., & Keefe, R. (1981). Effects of vestibular stimulation on spontaneous use of verbal language in developmentally delayed children. *American Journal of Occupational Therapy,* 35, 101-104.

Morris, S.E. (1982a). *The normal acquisition of feeding skills: Implications for assessment and treatment.* New York: Therapeutic Media.

Morris, S.E. (1982b). *Prespeech assessment scale.* Clifton, NJ: J.A. Preston.

Ottenbacher, K. (1978). Identifying vestibular processing dysfunction in learning disabled children. *American Journal of Occupational Therapy,* 32, 217-221.

Ray, T.C., King, L.J., & Grandin, T. (1988). The effectiveness of self-initiated vestibular stimulation in producing speech sounds in an autistic child. *The Occupational Therapy Journal of Research,* 8, 186-190.

Remling, D.D., (1990). The motor-language lab—A collaborative effort in the public schools. *Occupational Therapy Forum,* 26, 1-8.

Rider, B.A. (1974). Abnormal postural reflexes in dysphasic children. *American Journal of Occupational Therapy,* 28, 351-353.

Robinson, A.L. (1977). Play: The arena for acquisition of rules for competent behavior. *American Journal of Occupational Therapy,* 31, 248-253.

Schaff, R. (1985). The frequency of vestibular disorders in developmentally delayed preschoolers with otitis media. *American Journal of Occupational Therapy,* 39, 247-252.

Scharfenaker, S., Hickman, L., & Braden, M. (1991). An integrated approach to intervention. In R.J. Hagerman & A.C. Silverman (Eds.). *Fragile X syndrome: Diagnosis, treatment, and research* (pp.327-372). Baltimore, MD: Johns Hopkins University Press.

Sene, A., & Fisher, S. (1985). The value of combined occupational therapy and speech therapy in pediatrics. *British Journal of Occupational Therapy, 48,* 132-134.

Stilwell, J.M., Crowe, T.K., & McCallum, L.W. (1978). Postrotary nystagmus duration as a function of communication disorders. *American Journal of Occupational Therapy, 32,* 222-228.

Van Housen-Selley, K. (1987, Autumn). Insights into motor skills in fragile X syndrome. *The Fragile X Foundation Newsletter,* 2-3.

Weeks, Z.R. (1979a). Effects of the vestibular system on human development, Part 1: Overview of functions and effects of stimulation. *Journal of Occupational Therapy, 33,* 376-381.

Weeks, Z.R. (1979b). Effects of the vestibular system on human development, Part II: Effects of vestibular stimulation on mentally retarded, emotionally disturbed, and learning-disabled individuals. *American Journal of Occupational Therapy, 33,* 450-457.

Weiss-Lambrou, R., Tetreault, S., & Dudley, J. (1989). The relationship between oral sensation and drooling in persons with cerebral palsy. *American Journal of Occupational Therapy, 43,* 155-161.

Windeck, S.L., & Laurel, M. (1989). A theoretical framework combining speech-language therapy with sensory integration treatment. *Sensory Integration Special Interest Section Newsletter, 12,* 1-5.

ADDITIONAL READINGS

Bailey, D.M. (1978). Effects of vestibular stimulation on verbalizations in chronic schizophrenics. *American Journal of Occupational Therapy, 33,* 445-450.

Chu, S.K.H. (1991, September). Sensory integration and autism. *Sensory Integration Quarterly,* 3-6.

Domaracki, L.S., & Sisson, L.A. (1990). Decreasing drooling with oral motor stimulation in children with multiple disabilities. *American Journal of Occupational Therapy, 44,* 680-684.

Jenkins, E., & Lohr (1964). Severe articulation disorders and motor ability. *Journal of Speech and Hearing Disorders, 29,* 286-292.

Morrison, D., & Pothier (1972). Two different remedial training programs and the development of mentally retarded preschoolers. *American Journal of Mental Deficiency, 77,* 251-258.

Morrison, D., & Pothier. (1978). Effects of sensory-motor training on the language development of retarded preschoolers. *American Journal of Orthopsychiatry, 48,* 310-319.

Perozzi, A.J. (1972). Language acquisition as adaptive behavior. *Mental Retardation, 10,* 32-34.

PART IV

HOW HAVE WE APPLIED THESE TECHNIQUES?

9

A CASE STUDY

A case study at Ivymount school revealed impressive results using sensory integrative principles in delivering sensory motor and language treatment. Changes were observed in sensory processing, language, and overall functional level of a boy with fragile X. John's program at Ivymount is representative of the type of programming done with other fragile X students, and also with students who do not have fragile X but have similar needs in the areas of sensory integration, language, and academics.

BACKGROUND INFORMATION

John is a male student at Ivymount School. His birthdate is May 5, 1980. John entered Ivymount School in September 1987, at the age of 7 years, 4 months. He had previously been enrolled in a variety of placements in public school programs for multihandicapped children, in which he had difficulty receiving the intensity and integration of services he needed. He has a diagnosis of fragile X syndrome.

Ivymount School is a private school in Montgomery County, MD. The school was founded in 1961 as Christ Church Child Center as a program for children with mental retardation. Over the years, the population changed as the area's public schools began to increase programming options for special needs children. Today, Ivymount serves approximately 200 children from birth to 15 years of age. The majority of the children are categorized as "Multiply

Handicapped," although some tend to be primarily learning disabled or emotionally handicapped. Multiply handicapped, by the school's definition, means a child with a variety of communication, sensory motor, behavioral, and cognitive deficits that make it difficult for the child to be appropriately served in public school programs. The school has an intensive related service component: 12 speech-language therapists, 11 occupational therapists, 3 physical therapists, 5 social workers, a music therapist, an adaptive physical education teacher, and a computer specialist.

When he entered Ivymount, John exhibited many typical fragile X characteristics, including, in the sensory integration area, tactile defensiveness, poor tactile discrimination, decreased processing of vestibular input resulting in low muscle tone with decreased proximal stability, poor motor planning, gravitational insecurity, problems controlling emotional responses, problems with bilateral integration, lack of eye/hand coordination and inconsistent hand preference, presence of primitive postural reflexes, poor ocular-motor skills, decreased balance, olfactory and auditory hypersensitivity, hyperactivity, poor attending skills, self-stimulatory behaviors, and gross, fine, and perceptual motor delays.

In the language area, John exhibited rapid and perseverative speech, cluttering, poor pragmatic language skills, including poor eye contact, poor auditory processing skills, with relative strength in the single-word vocabulary area, and difficulty with sequencing.

His first teacher at Ivymount made the following notes to describe his classroom behavior:

> "difficulty attending, poor eye contact, gets out of seat frequently, appears anxious and tense, rubs face, shuts out stimuli by covering his eyes, lots of perseverative verbalizations, pitch and rate of speech are high, inappropriate stress and intonation patterns, tactile defensiveness, needs a carrel, teacher sometimes sits behind him to cut out distractions and allow attention only to her hands, needs calming techniques such as deep pressure, rocking, very patterned or organized activity, help with appropriate words, use of slow, whispered speech and gestures and signs."

He was referred to Ivymount School for an intensive, integrated special education program with particular emphasis on the foundation skills for academic achievement: language and sensory skills. It was recommended to the therapists at Ivymount that John receive combined occupational and speech-language therapies on a weekly basis. Therapies would focus on improved processing by combining vestibular and proprioceptive input with language and cognitive tasks and treat his sequencing and motor planning problems in a combined fashion.

Occupational therapy reports from John F. Kennedy Institute and a private practice (Bassin, 1986) indicated that John was unable to perform any of the Southern California Sensory Integration Test (Ayres, 1972), including Postrotary Nystagmus (PRN), before his admission to Ivymount. Problem areas listed were poor body awareness, overall gross and fine motor incoordination, and sensory integration dysfunction. Language evaluations done before John's admission revealed a child who had great difficulty performing on standardized tests. Observations by his previous speech-language pathologist were similar to those made by his first teacher at Ivymount.

At the time of his admission, results of the Brigance Inventory of Basic Skills (Brigance, 1983) indicated that John's gross motor skills scattered from the 2-year level to the 5-year, 6-month level, with an average score at the 3-year, 4-month level. His fine motor skills were at the 3-year level, with scattering up to the 5-year level. His Brigance language scores revealed performance at the 2- to 3-year level with strengths in vocabulary and body part knowledge. Other language tests done at this time were the Peabody Picture Vocabulary Test-Revised, Form L (Dunn & Dunn, 1981), on which John achieved an age equivalency of 5 years; the Token Test for Children (DiSimoni, 1978), on which he earned a standard score of 468 (mean = 500 ± 5), and Assigning Structural Stages (Miller, 1981), which placed John's syntactic skills at the 3 1/2- to 4-year level.

Classroom observations revealed a child who was not processing and integrating the sensory information in his environment. However, John showed good primary play skills and the ability to engage in imaginary play, motivation to learn, adaptability to the new school environment, good global memory, and potential for improved attending skills as seen by his ability to engage in simple sensory exploration tasks for long periods. Language strengths observed in the classroom included vocabulary, interest in a variety of topics, desire to interact socially, good general information, a sense of humor, and willingness to participate in role play.

OCCUPATIONAL THERAPY INTERVENTION

John was scheduled to receive OT for the 1987-88 school year at least two times a week. Therapeutic activities were selected with a focus on a sensory integrative and neurodevelopmental approach to enhance processing of sensory motor information and to promote academic learning. Treatment activities were designed to achieve these goals:

- John will discriminate and organize sensory input necessary for focusing on and attending to classroom and therapy lessons.
- John will demonstrate an awareness of body position and location in space while performing academic/therapy tasks involving stationary and dynamic positions.
- John will improve bilateral integration for efficiency and accuracy during movement and manipulative tasks in the classroom/therapy.

A more specific breakdown of these goals was developed as the 1987-88 Educational Management Plan. This directed the therapist to focus on increasing John' tolerance of tactile input, normalizing responses to vestibular input, assuming antigravity postures, focusing on pertinent visual information, improving auditory attending behavior, and normalizing reactions to olfactory input in the area of sensory processing. In other goal areas the focus was to be on an increased awareness of motoric function of his body parts, reaching across midline, and using one hand as a manipulator and the other as a stabilizer. A therapist checklist was written, with items selected for observation and measurement of progress and change. Areas included were performance levels on test items, treatment performance, and classroom performance. Also, a physical therapy consultation was initiated on an as-needed basis. Since John's academic picture was so affected by his sensory integrative dysfunction, treatment was primarily designed to facilitate optimal processing in all sensory modes. The following plan of action was initiated:

1. Improve vestibular processing by providing movement experiences with a motor response in a variety of positions using suspended equipment and scooter boards.
2. Improve tactile processing by providing firm tactile input with various lotions, brushes, and vibrators, plus providing activities requiring tactile exploration and discrimination.
3. Decrease abnormal olfactory self-stimulation through self-directed olfactory and gustatory stimulation activities. Sensory input experiences were chosen using natural input without artificial additives, with qualities and quantities controlled by the therapist.

4. Improve muscle tone through vestibular activities as well as jumping, climbing, work on the therapy ball, and positioning to improve individual muscle groups. Focus on the abdominal and trunk muscles first.
5. Improve crossing midline in activities through use of both upper extremities together and in a variety of different patterns against both sides of the body.

As the above areas improved, activities were selected that involved motor planning and bilateral coordination. When John was overstimulated, inhibitory techniques with a calming affect on his behavior were incorporated into the classroom and therapy situations as needed.

Service Delivery

John was seen for direct services once a week individually for 30 minutes and one time weekly with the speech therapist in the OT clinic for another 30 minutes. The individual sessions were primarily self-directed sensory integration treatment activities, and the combined OT and language sessions consisted of purposeful sensory motor activities designed to facilitate increased sensory processing and pragmatic skills. He also participated in a weekly functional group co-led by the SLP and OT, with such activities as "sensory integration cooking," gardening, art, and gross motor play. The use of combined treatment techniques is dealt with in another section of this chapter. Indirect services included classroom observation and consultation, weekly team planning meetings for curriculum development, and regular inservicing for other professionals and parents to increase their understanding of how a sensory integration framework operates. John was also seen on an as-needed basis for emergency intervention with calming techniques designed to ameliorate stress. These additional therapy sessions were short and intense and often co-led by the teacher. Initially in the school year the interventions were conducted almost daily; eventually this tapered off because of changes in John's functional level and teacher education. Therapy equipment such as a cloud, bean bag chair, weighted vest, or blanket for rolling up in were placed in the classroom as needed for calming purposes. Other equipment such as balls, rolls, scooter boards, and barrels were available for loan to the classroom for facilitating gross motor play.

SPEECH AND LANGUAGE THERAPY INTERVENTION

John's Individual Education Plan specified at least 60 minutes per week of speech and language therapy. Treatment activities were selected to improve his language-use abilities for better functioning in a variety of settings. The following goals were identified:

- John will improve his ability to process auditory information.
- John will improve social use of language.
- John will improve his ability to organize and express a coherent message.
- John will improve receptive and expressive knowledge of specific language concepts.
- John will improve oral sensory motor skills for eating and speech.
- John will improve intelligibility of speech.

These objectives were broken down into more specific interim goals that could be measured behaviorally. The classroom teachers and occupational therapist were partners in the speech and language intervention. John's problems with language influenced every part of his day, including his difficulty with transitions and with waiting his turn. His poor attention and topic maintenance and his perseverative, sometimes unintelligible, speech impeded his development of social relationships in his new school, also making it difficult for him to use language as a behavioral intervention technique during out-of-control episodes. The specific goals addressed by the speech-language pathologist were:

1. Improve auditory processing by providing practice in following routine two-part directions with visual cues, by teaching the meaning of "where" and "how many" questions, and by attending to and labeling a variety of environmental sounds.
2. Improve social language by increasing eye contact, improving conversational turn-taking, teaching appropriate ways to gain attention, and reducing perseverative, noncommunicative utterances.
3. Improve expressive language organization by helping him relate personal, experiential events using logical sequence and appropriate amount of detail.

4. Improve concept knowledge by teaching the meaning of quantitative and size concepts (more, as many, long, short, tall) and spatial concepts (in front, behind, next to, beside).
5. Improve oral sensory-motor skills by normalizing sensitivity in the oral area, and designing a program of stimulation activities to promote adequate mobility of the tongue, lips, and jaw.
6. Improve speech intelligibility by appropriate use of suprasegmentals such as rate, stress, and fluency.

Service Delivery

John was seen by the SLP once a week individually, once in combined speech and language-occupational therapy, and in the classroom for weekly language group, language-functional group (co-led by the SLP and OT), and a daily "language breakfast" led once a week by the SLP and by the teachers the other 4 days. The guiding principles of every language activity were that it be experiential, high-interest, and incorporate a sensory motor component. Visual cues and a predictable, gestalt-oriented approach were also employed. Sign language and pictures were used to support auditory input throughout the day. Role play was used extensively for practice of social routines, questions, concepts, and academics. The emphasis was always on integration of skills. For example, the daily language breakfast incorporated oral sensory motor exercises (preparatory stimulation, varying food textures, and utensil use), social language (asking for things, saying thank you, body orientation), concepts (more, full, big, small), and academics (counting cups, 1:1 correspondence). In addition, breakfast food was frequently student-prepared, to address fine motor and visual motor skills, as well as help reduce sensory defensiveness.

Combined speech and language/occupational therapy provided the best examples of integrated service. One activity that was very successful with John was a sequencing activity built on the steps in getting ready for school in the morning. When baseline data was collected, John was unable to describe this sequence, even with toy items available as prompts. He perseverated on one activity—the car coming out of the garage—and was unable to move on. His perseveration led him to verbally and motorically express increasingly inappropriate activities involving the car and garage, eventually putting all the toy household items, including the toilet, into the garage. The sessions took place in the OT suite with suspended equipment available. Using OT equipment, areas were set up to simulate a bedroom, bathroom, eating area, and car.

The sequence being taught was getting ready for school in the morning. It began with John in "bed"—an innertube—being held firmly in a flexed position to calm him. He then "woke up" and climbed through an OT-constructed door to the "bathroom," where a toothbrush and shaving cream were used to provide input to his face, mouth, and hands. As it was done firmly, John tolerated this well. Getting dressed was next, using a heavy weighted coat for more deep pressure. John then progressed to the "breakfast table," a barrel on which he could weight shift and receive vestibular and proprioceptive input. As the speech-language therapist worked on questions and classification tasks (with pictures of foods), the OT facilitated crossing midline and providing vestibular input by rocking. John also was allowed to really eat some fruit for additional sensory stimulation and practice of biting and chewing.

The final step in the story was the "car," a suspended flexion disc swing that provided vestibular input as he worked on the auditory-visual processing task of answering the speech-language therapist's questions by choosing the correct picture. Specific language goals in this activity included sequencing, classifying items, and answering questions. OT goals included motor planning, increasing tone through vestibular input, crossing midline, increasing calm and attentive behavior through deep tactile and proprioceptive input, and decreasing defensiveness to tactile input in the face and hands.

EDUCATIONAL PROGRAM

John's daily academic groups, reading, math, and visual/fine-motor, were designed to teach specific skills at his level, with constant attention to the need for sensory components to calm and organize him. Attention was paid to positioning John where he was least likely to feel crowded by other children. The teachers avoided excessive eye contact in their interactions with John, often sitting behind or beside him. A carrel was often used to block distractions. In the classroom, a sensory box (see Chapter 6) was always available. Before activities requiring sustained attention, such as listening to a story, a sensory stimulation time was held using lotion, brushes, and deep pressure for calming. Seating in supportive chairs, with Dysem on the seats and a seatbelt, provided stabilization. Light, noise, and movement were controlled as much as possible, especially at the beginning of the year. The staff kept verbal reinforcement and praise low-key, and often visual rewards (such as a star) were given with little or no verbal accompaniment.

John participated in varied structured play activities designed to encourage development of cognitive skills and language, and to teach the children in a structured way how to progress in their imaginative play level during their own spontaneous interactions. These situations were tied into a weekly theme and other lesson plans. For instance, a play activity about going to the grocery store would be paired with a field trip to the store and a circle time focusing on food groups. Preacademic goals such as counting, matching, classification, and sequencing were frequently addressed in the play sessions.

John also participated in music therapy and adaptive physical education with his class on a weekly basis. These activities were designed to facilitate integration of sensory processing and skill development in age-appropriate activities.

PROGRESS

Brigance testing completed in January 1988 revealed that John's gross motor skills scattered from the 2-year level to the 7-year level, with an average score at the 4-year level. His fine motor skills were solidly at the 3-year level, with scattering to the 5-year level. John's performance had improved in the areas of walking, stair climbing, running, kicking, balance, and catching and bouncing a ball. No significant changes were made in fine motor skills.

By April of that school year, the following comments were made about his progress in OT:

> "He is able to participate in a five minute art or cooking activity which involves touch without asking to wash his hands in the middle. He is initiating and participating in swinging activities without becoming overstimulated for longer periods of time. John no longer covers his eyes and only inappropriately smells objects when stressed out. The use of his body continues to be a puzzle for John; however, he will readily explore how to do a task in a play situation. John requires less handling to facilitate crossing the midline, but still cannot do it consistently without this support."

John showed many gains in language skills by the spring of 1988. Although he continued to require some external cues and organizing strategies to remain calm and attentive in group activities, John demonstrated very appropriate eye contact and much improved initiation and interaction skills. He was able to tell the story—or events—of a complete activity (with pictures) on request. He enjoyed telling jokes to peers and teachers. Formal testing indicated 1- to 2-years progress in his comprehension of single words and language forms.

CONCLUSION

John has continued his educational and therapeutic program at Ivymount. To this day, his program continues to change and evolve, reflecting his needs and facilitating optimal growth in language, sensory integration, motor skills, and functional abilities.

John's therapists and teachers feel that John has learned a great deal through his program at Ivymount. His improved ability to function calmly in a classroom setting was dramatic during the first year and has continued. John has also been a teacher. Development of his program helped us pull together, document, and expand on integrated treatment activities we had been implementing on a less formal and consistent basis for a long time. In a sense, John's treatment plan was the seed that eventually grew into this book.

REFERENCES

Ayres, A.J. (1972). *Southern California sensory integration test.* Los Angeles: Western Psychological Services.

Bassin, B. (1986). Occupational therapy report.

Brigance, A.H. (1983). *Brigance inventory of basic skills.* North Billerica, MA: Curriculum Associates, Inc.

DiSimoni, F. (1978). *The token test for children.* Boston: Teaching Resources Corporation.

Dunn, L.M., & Dunn, L.M. (1981). *Peabody picture vocabulary test—revised.* Circle Pines, MN: American Guidance Service.

Miller, J.F. (1981). Assigning structural stages. In Miller, J.F. (Ed.), *Assessing language production in children* (pp. 31-36). Baltimore: University Park Press.

APPENDIX A

PEOPLE AND PLACES TO CONTACT

For more information about fragile X syndrome, these organizations and individuals may be helpful.

ORGANIZATION

The National Fragile X Foundation
1441 York St., Suite 215
Denver, CO 80206
1-800-688-8765

NATIONAL FRAGILE X FOUNDATION RESOURCE CENTERS

University of South Alabama
Department of Medical Genetics
Room 214, CCCB
Mobile, AL 36688
(250) 460-7500

Medical Genetics Department
Children's Hospital Medical
Center
747 52nd St.
Oakland, CA 94609
(415) 428-3550

North Los Angeles County
Resource Center
8353 Sepulveda Blvd.
Sepulveda, CA 91343
(818) 895-5316

Medical Genetics
Emory University School of
Medicine
2040 Ridgewood Dr.
Atlanta, GA 30322
(404) 727-5840

National Fragile X Association of America
PO Box 39
Parkridge, IL 60063

Kennedy Institute Behavioral Genetics
Research Center
707 N. Broadway
Baltimore, MD 21205
(301) 550-9913

Oakland County Mental Health
Services
1200 North Telegraph
Pontiac, MI 48053
(313) 858-1225

Morristown Memorial Hospital
DDC, Box 60
Morristown, NJ 07960
(201) 285-4095

Fragile X Association of New York
61 Dean St.
Brooklyn, NY 11201
(718) 875-4901

Duke University Medical Center
Box 3364
Durham, NC 27710
(919) 684-5513

Fragile X Association of Oregon, Inc.
7205 SE 32nd Ave.
Portland, OR 97202
(503) 774-7167

Department of Pediatrics
Medical College of Ohio
PO Box 10008
Toledo, OH 43699
(419) 381-4435

Genetic Center
One Children's Plaza
Dayton, OH 45404
(513) 226-8408

People of Color
PO Box 1952
Cleveland, OH 44106
(216) 751-8734

Fragile X Program
Albert Einstein Medical Center
5501 Old York Rd.
Philadelphia, PA 19141-3098
(215) 456-6786

The Neighborhood Program
4908 Danby Dr.
Nashville, TN 37211
(615) 834-2137

Academic Learning Clinic
SW Texas State University
San Marcos, TX 78666-4616
(512) 245-2157

Fragile X Program
University of Washington
CDMRC-WJ-10
Seattle, WA 98195
(206) 685-3205

Parent Resource Center
Laramie County School Dist #11
2810 House Ave.
Cheyenne, WY 82001
(307) 771-2172

Lakehead Fragile X Resource
Center
354 Munro St.
Thunderbay, ONT P7A 2N5
Canada
(807) 343-4253

Developmental Counseling
Service
Ongwanada
191 Portsmouth Ave.
Kingston, ONT K7M 8A6
Canada (613) 548-4417

AUDIO-VISUAL RESOURCES

Audio recordings of conference proceedings: First National Fragile X
Conference, Denver, CO, December 1987. Contact Expectations Unlim-
ited, Inc., P.O. Box 655, Niwot, CO 80542.

Audio recordings of conference proceedings: After the Diagnosis, Then What? Life with the Fragile X Child, at Home and at School, Baltimore, MD, November, 1989. Contact Chesapeake Audio/Visual Communications, 6330 Howard Lane, Elkridge, MD 21227. (301) 796-0040; Fax (301) 379-0812.

Audio recordings of conference proceedings: First Southeastern Regional Conference on Fragile X Syndrome, Durham, NC, December 1988. Available from Dr. Gail Spirodigliozzo, 1-800-654-FRAX.

Video: Fragile X Syndrome: Diagnosis and Treatment. Available from National Fragile X Foundation, 1441 York St., Suite 215, Denver, CO 80206. Attn: Sabrina Jewell-Smart.

Video: Fragile X Syndrome: Family Perspectives. Available from Co-ordinator, Developmental Counseling Service, Ongwanada, Penrose Division, 752 King St., West Kingston, Ontario, Canada 613-544-9611, ext. 266.

Video: What is Fragile X Syndrome? by Dr. Ave Lachiewicz. Available from Pam Brode, Fragile X Southeast Network, Duke University Medical Center, Box 3364, Durham, NC 27710. 919-684-5513.

Video: Genetic Counseling Issues by Amy Cronister, M.S. Taped at First Southeastern Regional Conference on Fragile X Syndrome, Durham, NC, December 1988. Available from Ave Lachiewicz, M.D., Duke University Medical Center, Child Development Unit, Box 3364, Durham, NC 27710.

Video: CBS's 48 Hours: Fragile X Syndrome. Available from CBS, 1-800-338-4847.

Index